CW00495643

Extreme Rapid Weight Loss Hypnosis

for Women

Weight Loss With Self-Hypnosis and Meditation.
Increase Your Self-Esteem
and Start Being Kind to Yourself.

ROSE ALLEN

—
5

Introduction

Hypnosis for weight loss is basically using hypnosis techniques to allow you to lose weight. It is a way to shed a few extra pounds. But most of the time, it is paired with a diet plan. You should continue a good regimen of food, followed by moderate exercise. But this will allow you to lose weight faster, and if you are a person who has cravings for things, then this will help you immensely.

Once you understand the practice and how it is conducted, you will find that everything makes sense. Hypnosis works for weight loss because of the relationship between our minds and bodies. Without proper communication being relayed from our minds to our bodies, we would not be able to function correctly. Since hypnosis allows the brain to adopt new ideas and habits, it can help push anyone in the right direction and could potentially improve our quality of living.

It is also a part of the counseling that some people get. You will be able to get help on your issues regarding food, and this form of hypnosis will allow you to have a better time with your cravings. You can do this with a professional, but you can also do it on your own. It will let you have control of your life, and you will control those bad cravings you have.

How it works is simple. When you are using hypnosis, you are in a state of absorption and concentration. You are also in a very relaxed and suggestible state, so whatever is said to you is taken in a literal manner. You will use mental images to convey the meaning of the words that are spoken. You will have your attention focused on that, and when your mind is in a state of concentration, you will start to have your subconscious handle your cravings. It is a remarkable way to keep yourself in check so you will be able to lose a few extra pounds while still trying to keep your body in shape. It is most ideal if you do this with a diet and exercise routine, for it will allow you to get through it better and achieve more results.

With hypnosis for weight loss, you will allow yourself to handle your body in a positive manner. If you do this, you will actually allow yourself to control your cravings and desires through the use of hypnosis. It might seem crazy, but it is possible. It's a great way to take life by the horns. By doing this, you'll be able to allow yourself the benefit of controlling the factors in your life, such as stress or how much you eat, and turning them around to give yourself a more positive image that will benefit you in ways you've never expected before.

You will be guided on how you can achieve the maximum benefits of hypnosis and hypnotherapy for weight loss. So, without further ado, let's turn the page and learn the secrets of hypnosis.

Chapter 1. What is Hypnosis?

Hypnosis is a state of inner absorption; concentration also concentrated focus. It is comparable to getting a magnifying glass to focus the rays of the sun and make them more powerful. Alike, when our minds are concentrated and focused, we are prepared to use our minds more ardently. Because hypnosis allows people to use more of their possible, knowing self-hypnosis is the very best activity of self-control.

Hypnosis is a method or set of methods that allow the body and brain to share information better. One of those methods is called a trance. It is a process of creating an inner-self experience of focused consciousness that permits your own body and head to take and talk about your goals, beliefs, and expectations as precise. The targeted goal of your comprehension magnifies your own energy of understanding (and also the capacity of your knowledge) to make your subconscious mind to act and take upon a target.

Hypnosis is a mental phenomenon. The therapies revolving around and based on hypnosis have a significant advantage over other forms of treatment. While medicine consumption and doctor sessions may help a patient recover from life troubles, hypnosis doesn't require so much of hassle. All one has to do is sit quietly in the company of hypnotic assistance, and you are good to go. The best part about hypnosis is that it deals with everything mental and rarely requires any physical effort to be put in for it to succeed.

To a lot of people, hypnosis is a very esoteric concept that has little practical use in daily living. It is magic, something practiced by higher beings, maybe something that doesn't even exist, or something that only exists in fantasy. Little do most people know, hypnosis is actually a part of our daily lives, whether we realize it or not. Self-talk is the things we tell ourselves internally and externally. The things we say like "I am ugly," "I am stupid," "You could've done this or that better," "They will never love you,"—these are hypnotic phrases that program our mind in ways we take for granted. The practice of hypnosis is merely becoming aware of the power we have over our own thoughts and honing it, grabbing hold of it like a wild beast, taming it, taking control of it, and using it to do what we want it to do.

To get more specific, hypnosis involves honing the will, of the focus and attention, and, therefore, intention of the subject. The subject is the one who is being hypnotized. Generally, the subject and the practitioner are two separate people. The practitioner can be a magician. I'm sure you've seen one at the state fair or the amusement park asking for volunteers, but in more practical terms, the practitioner can be a licensed clinical therapist. This is because hypnotism can have a potent effect on the betterment of the subject. Therapists often use hypnotism to break down barriers in the psyche and address problems head-on in ways that can't be done through a simple conversation, methods that are traditionally blocked by the conscious, protecting the sub-conscious. But, alas, the practitioner and the subject can most importantly be the same person. You can perform hypnosis on yourself and for your own betterment. It involves a solid understanding of the patterns of the conscious and subconscious mind and a keen awareness of where your mind goes and what it is focusing on at any given time.

Traditionally, hypnosis involves the summoning of a relaxed, almost trance-like state—a state where the conscious mind is less guarded over what comes and goes from its sub-conscious brother. This can be achieved in a large, almost infinite number of ways. Once a state of relaxation is achieved, simple core concepts are introduced, or extracted from, the sub-conscious mind, depending on the intended effect the hypnosis is to have.

Besides false memories that can be implanted for positive goals, such as this, real memories that have been repressed by the conscious mind can be extracted; a big reason clinical practitioners practice hypnosis. Hypnosis gets to the core of past trauma. This will come into play later as we realize the power hypnosis can have on changing ingrained patterns of behavior that we have learned and developed over time that negatively affect us in one way or another in our daily living, which will come to be the most significant point this will make.

Besides the concept of implanting or detracting false and real memories, a very simple practice of hypnosis involves the implantation of simple positive core concepts that positively benefit the core beings—things as simple as saying, "I am loved," or "I am not stupid," or "I can do this." Post-hypnotic suggestions are the clinical term for these phrases when induced to the subject after achieving what is called the hypnotic state, or trance state, the desired state of relaxation is the one that strives for in hypnosis. This is another very powerful concept in hypnosis. When practiced on the self, these positive phrases can be repeated over and over. These affirmations will be known to us as "mantras." This is a word to remember here.

Chapter 2. Where is Hypnotism Utilized

The use of Hypnosis is boundless in nature. The most widely recognized are weight and smoking control. It can likewise be utilized to liquor abuse, drug compulsion, stress, and different other mental issues, for example, sadness and impulse. Spellbinding can also be used to create a memory, expand the focus, and enhance study propensities and test-taking. It can likewise help improve fearlessness and upgrade athletic capacities. Right away, spellbinding is being utilized viably as a part of a wide range of settings, including instructive, therapeutic, dental, and legitimate territories and in sales.

The differences between the art of hypnotism and other mental action lie in the features of hypnotism. In the parts below, we explore the various facets of hypnotism.

One of the most prominent features of hypnotism is that it deals with the mind and opens the gates of it. It enhances your mental stability and strength. You will be gaining more focus, and you will concentrate better. When you take a few moments to strategize and rethink your decisions every day, you will be able to make better decisions. With mental enhancement comes the benefit of increasing your memory. The process of hypnotism works by getting rid of any unwanted distractions. It removes blocks in memories by filtering out your thoughts and makes information more accessible in our heads. With the use of hypnosis, you can be able to control your life a lot better. It prevents you from doing unnecessary tasks and breaks down your schedule to fit in only the important functions. It reduces addiction to certain things. For instance, through hypnotism, you can reduce the addiction to smoking. It also makes you more focused and goal-oriented. The mind is trained to only focus on the necessities. You can control your reactions and responses due to an increase in clarity. This will enhance your interpersonal skills. With hypnosis, you will be able to reduce bad habits and break addictions. These can range from mild addictions like coffee addictions or nail-biting to severe addictions like smoking. There are many cases where bad habits start to get restored. This is prevented by hypnotism. You can control your behavior, and because of this, you can keep the qualities that you like in yourself and discard those that you feel the need to change. Hypnotism is attributed to positive transformation. It gives you a new direction and a new perspective towards things. When combined with NLP, you are able to broaden your horizons and make way for new experiences. With you being more in control, your self-esteem increases, and you grow. As you get out of unhealthy habits and behavioral traits, you will find better things to focus on. You will stop to think with your emotions and think practically instead. It keeps you healthy and happy. It also increases your problem-solving skills.

Here is a simple list of the different situations where hypnosis can be of great help:

1. As most of the reasons why people undergo hypnosis are the following:

2. Change habits and behaviors such as smoking, smoking, or hair-pulling on.

3. Heal anxiety disorders or ailments

4. Detect subconscious emotional struggles or dynamics that underlie many different symptoms.

5. Alleviate pain.

6. Supply anesthesia throughout the surgery.

7. Assist wounds in healing quicker.

8. Heal skin disorders.

9. Heal the irritable bowel syndrome.

10. Provide relief for allergies.

11. Encourage the healing of asthma.

12. Curb or boost the immune system.

13. Address several different applications, like expediting weight-loss.

14. The treatment of ongoing agony conditions, for example, rheumatoid joint pain

15. The therapy and decrease of agony during labor

16. The reduction in the side effects of dementia

17. The reduction of sickness and regurgitating in patients experiencing chemotherapy

18. Control of anger and mode swings during dental strategies

19. Disposal of skin conditions including moles and psoriasis

20. Lightening of side effects related to peevish entrail condition

21. Eating Disorders can be treated as well as problems associated with weight.

22. Stress Disorders – In other words those problems of a health nature that can be treated by stress control – i.e., high blood pressure

23. Panic attacks

24. Gastrointestinal problems that are affected by a nervous disposition.

25. Habits such as smoking and those that relate to addiction.

26. Lack of Confidence can relate to embarrassment both in the workplace and socially.

27. Fears & Phobias: Many phobias affect people, and these may not necessarily be logical ones. People are scared of a variety of things.

28. Psycho-sexual issues such as impotence or being worried about sexual performance.

29. Speech impediments.

30. Problems that relate to traumatic experiences and these can include unresolved issues arising from death, loss, etc.

31. Gynecological problems such as heavy periods, menopause trauma.

32. Study problems – People with a lack of confidence may fail exams even if they know their study work.

33. Pain – Hypnosis can help people deal with long term pain management.

34. Long term and serious illness management, such as in cases of AIDS, cancer, and M.S.

So, why an individual chooses to attempt Hypnosis? At times, individuals may search out Hypnosis to help manage ceaseless torment or to mitigate pain and uneasiness brought about by clinical techniques, for example, medical procedure or labor. Hypnosis has additionally been utilized to help individuals with conduct changes, for example, stopping smoking, getting more fit, or forestalling bed-wetting.

Other Truths About Hypnosis

1. Hypnosis is complex and requires tons of sessions as well as schooling.
2. For a person to experience hypnosis, it must be done by someone who understands just how to take action to you.
3. One loses consciousness after getting a hypnotic trance.
4. The subconscious mind won't be able to tell differences between what is imagined and what is real.
5. Hypnosis has the ability to make a person do things that are contrary to a will or split your own worth.
6. Many women and men enter trance daily.
7. Your body communicates with its own language.
8. It's likely to use hypnosis to affect your physical responses, such as breathing .digestion, etc.
9. Medical hypnosis is equal or the same as stage hypnosis
10. Most of the time, the person is not aware that they are in a trance.
11. Hypnosis is a just psychological or psychological phenomenon; it is "all in the mind "
12. Some several women and men can't be hypnotized.
13. With hypnosis, you're going to have the ability to brings signals and messages to the whole body, and your body may provide you messages.

Ways to Practice Hypnosis

1. Hypnosis in Therapy

A session directed by a hypnotist and one customer. The main issue with hypnotherapy is that most states have very few if any, laws overseeing the usage of entrancing in a remedial or clinical setting. To discover a legal or legit individual in your general state contact the National Guild of Hypnotists, you will be given the names of a few guaranteed hypnotists in your general state. Communicate those people and verify you are OK with the individual before setting up a session.

2. Group Hypnosis

Normally led in a gathering session with the end goal of:

- A self-improvement session to lessen the harmful habits of a person: quit smoking, learning self-hypnosis, and so on. Not as good as a one-on-one session, in any case, but less expensive.

3. Self-Hypnosis

This is a type of hypnosis that you can do at home or wherever you feel like to control yourself from triggers that surround you. When a man takes in the self-hypnosis process, he/she can keep on using it as a device to achieve numerous positive changes. This can be used for simple cases rather than complicated ones.

4. Hypnosis CDs and Downloads

This method is much ideal for those individuals who don't have ample time in setting schedules for self-Hypnosis or a one-on-one session with a therapist. A CD or Download can be listened to at the time he/she is about to sleep, and this method can be effective when used properly and when done habitually.

Chapter 3. Hypnotherapy and Hypnosis

Hypnosis and hypnotherapy are often described as being one in the same practice, but they are not. Hypnotherapy is a technique used by hypnotists to treat a subject's concern or problem. In this kind of situation, the subconscious mind is more accessible where habits, memory, and emotions are located, which allows the hypnotist to aid and guide a subject to achieve long-lasting and positive changes in their lives. Hypnotherapy is a kind of guided hypnosis that mainly focuses on concentration, while hypnosis refers to the act of guiding an individual into a trance state of mind. With hypnosis, this state is commonly referred to as either a resting state of relaxation, induced suggestibility, or hyper-focus.

Something the average student or individual working battles with every day is to keep focus during their daily routine. A consistent lack of focus may leave an individual feeling tired, unmotivated, stressed, and inefficient. That's just one of the main reasons why hypnotherapy serves as the ultimate solution for anyone looking to improve productivity, relieve stress and anxiety, and boost their overall health.

Hypnotherapy is used in various instances, all of which have been proven to be very effective. It is similar to other types of psychological treatments with benefits that are similar to those of psychotherapy.

The practice treats conditions, including phobias, anxiety disorders, bad habits, weight gain, substance abuse, learning disorders, poor communication skills, and can even treat pain. It can resolve digestive and gastrointestinal disorders, as well as severe hormonal skin disorders, aiding as a massive solution to many different issues people face daily and are often unaware of how to treat.

Many patients with immune disorders or severe conditions, such as cancer, can also be treated with hypnotherapy as it is known for its pain-relieving abilities. It is especially helpful and used when patients undergo chemotherapy or physical rehabilitation that is excessively painful.

Hypnotherapy is carried out by a therapist in a therapeutic and tranquil environment that allows the patient to enter and remain in a focused state of mind. Apart from its incredible benefits, it can adjust the mind and shift mental behavior, almost tricking the brain into focusing on positive intentions. Often, with severe cases, such as advanced stages of cancer, patients are almost convinced that they are not going to live very long. Some may even receive their expected date of passing from their medical practitioner.

Faced with extreme negativity, such as a patient being told that they are going to die, patients tend to give up.

Now, regardless of what you believe, what your mind conceives to believe may very well become a reality. This manner of thinking holds a lot of truth and could set a patient apart from surviving their condition. Although it is difficult to achieve a state of mind where one is positive when faced with illness, hypnotherapy can indeed adjust one's thought process and retrain the brain into thinking only positive thoughts.

In essence, a cancer patient's attitude can massively contribute to their probability of healing. Hypnotherapy can, in fact, relieve not only pain but also add a mental shield against negative thinking processes that could contribute to a patient's inability to recover.

From various types of recovery, acting as more than just a supportive release for pain, emotional and mental stability, something many individuals find fascinating is that one can lose weight with hypnotherapy.

Depending on how severe the problem being treated is, hypnotherapy may take longer to see a difference. Upon meeting with a hypnotherapist, the practitioner will assess the extent of hypnotherapy required, measured in hours, for the patient to obtain the result they would like to see at the end of their course of therapy. A specific total number of hours will be prescribed to the patient, forming a part of alternative healthcare.

Take it as a tip, with hypnotherapy, and it is very important to feel comfortable with your practitioner, which is why you must seek out several just to find the right one. With hypnotherapy, it's always a good idea to ask around for recommendations and not settle for the first therapist you come across.

Since you now have a good understanding of hypnotherapy, it's necessary also to be informed about hypnosis.

Hypnosis refers to placing an individual in a trance state of mind, also referred to as deep relaxation, increased suggestibility, and hyper-focus.

Thinking about the different references related to hypnosis, one may think of it as being focused based on deep sleep. When we sleep, we tend to enter and exit a trance state quite often. This can also occur when we listen to music or when we are focused on reading a book or watching a movie. It invites a state of mind where our thought processes almost come to a halt as we are focused, and our brain suddenly even more so than it is used to. Whenever you immerse yourself into something and focus, you enter a trance state of mind.

So, what's the difference between professional hypnosis, the actual act of induced hypnosis, and our brief everyday moments of intense focus? Well, about the only difference is that with hypnosis, you are assisted with a hypnotherapist to enter a trance state of mind where you can achieve wonderful things. You can achieve a state of motivation, positivity, healing, stress-relief, and even weight loss.

The Myths:

Those who believe in myths or are superstitious have painted a picture of hypnosis that has managed to scare people away.

Whether you've heard about hypnosis in the media, saw it in a movie, or were shunned by your parents against learning more about it, you can rest assured that it's not as bad as society makes it out to be.

Can hypnotists control the minds of their patients? Of course not. Hypnosis is used as a medical practice to either relieve symptoms associated with pain, anxiety or help people to lose weight and get back on the healthy train again. It doesn't leave you feeling helpless or unaware of what you're doing.

During hypnotherapy, patients are still conscious and can hear everything that is happening around them, which is another reason why it is considered an entirely safe practice. To assure people, even more, it is next to impossible for anyone to be unconscious when undergoing hypnosis.

Differentiating between hypnosis and hypnotherapy, you now have learned that both practices have a similar foundation yet can help patients achieve different goals. Both practices can indeed help patients lose weight.

When you want to lose weight, you have to focus on different things. Losing weight is never just about cleaning up your diet and incorporating exercise into your daily routine.

Since stress is a major part of the reason why our bodies hold onto weight, hypnosis serves as the perfect solution to relieve stress and can also manage disorders, often contributing to weight gain. This includes both anxiety and depression. Additionally, it can help individuals with either an overactive or underactive thyroid to reach some level of balance, allowing one's body to lose weight permanently and sustainably. Hypnotherapy, on the other hand, is perfect for treating many different cases, including bad habits like smoking and overeating, which can contribute to a variety of eating disorders. Both can help you develop a bad relationship with food and even act as a means of coping with stress. That is why hypnosis and hypnotherapy can work hand-in-hand to achieve attainable results, depending on your needs. Hypnotherapy also relieves mind-body illnesses and reduces symptoms, including irritable bowel syndrome, skin conditions, and various types of addictions.

Unless you suffer from severe stress-related disorders that require you to engage in both practices, hypnotherapy can serve all of your needs concerning weight loss. It is the perfect option for anyone aiming to achieve long-term results.

Given that every decision, thought, and intention is birthed in mind, it's quite simple to see why hypnotherapy can solve a lot of the problems we as humans face with our bodies today.

Both hypnosis and hypnotherapy serve as practices that help deplete negative habits and can assist anyone, no matter how sick or unmotivated, to get back on track, follow a healthy diet, and attainable exercise program, as well as kick many harmful addictions.

Chapter 4. Frequently Asked Questions About Hypnosis

There are many myths, misconceptions, and fears surrounding hypnotism. These fears and misunderstandings are truly unfortunate because this is why many people reject or avoid hypnosis entirely when it could be of great help to them. Here are some common questions that people have that will be answered here directly.

Is Hypnosis Dangerous?

No. hypnotism is not dangerous. You need to ask for permission to the person when performing hypnosis on them, but at no time during the process will the person be in danger. At least not more than they are in regular everyday life. Hypnotism involves going into a deeply relaxed and focused state. The person does not lose consciousness or enter into another alternate reality where they have no control. In fact, they are still very aware and very much in control of themselves. The conscious mind is relaxed in this state so they will feel free of judgment and criticism. Some people fear that they will become weak or lose their own will to do things; this does not occur. You will also not share secrets or other things you would like to keep private unknowingly. The subject is always in the driver's seat.

Can You Secretly Hypnotize Someone?

This is something very common right now. If you Google hypnotism, all sorts of results come up about how to covertly or secretly hypnotize people. Now that you understand that hypnotism uses several states of mind that we commonly feel throughout the day and that it involves skillful communication, you may understand how false it is to "secretly" or "covertly" hypnotize someone. In essence, what these people are teaching are tools in relating to people and communication strategies that focus someone's attention, or distract them, or inspire certain emotional responses. These are things we do every day. Great speakers and leaders have mastered how to inspire and motivate and move people. Is that hypnotism? Well, not really. A movie or a book may have you so absorbed that you feel lost in it. Is that hypnotism?

You zone out and fantasize about the train going to work. In a sense, you are in a type of trance. Is that hypnotism? Well, many people will say that these are experiences within hypnotism, but it's an overstatement to say you are "hypnotized" in any sense of the word. So, can you secretly or covertly hypnotize someone? The question that lies under this is fear. A fear that someone can make me do something I don't want to do. Or can I make someone do something they don't want to do with these techniques? The answer is no. When you are completely absorbed in a film, do you spontaneously do something that is completely out of character? Of course not, you feel a stronger connection to your own experience, in fact. Have you ever been in such a daze going to work where you suddenly did something you deeply regretted later? Probably not. Being in a deep state of relaxation mentally and physically, and being highly suggestible doesn't change your morality.

Can You Turn Someone Bad Using Hypnosis?

Once again, no. The person's morality and propensity to do good or bad does not change. If, however, the person already has a propensity to do malicious or illegal things, they may. This is not due to the hypnosis, though, and rather it's related to how they are as people. If someone had the intention to turn another person into a horrible killing machine, they would not be able to use hypnosis to do so. Because at the subconscious level, the person would reject it as an immoral act. Being hypnotized doesn't turn you into a blank slate upon which you may be written, or raw clay that can be molded into whatever the instigator desires. There is a constant characteristic of the person that will always remain. You will never do something out of character. So then how does it work for good suggestions? Why would we accept a positive one rather than a negative or destructive suggestion? Because people naturally seek positivity. Yes, there are exceptions because there are people who don't, but this is an extremely minute percentage of the population. Generally, people are goal-oriented and seek wellness and will move towards life-giving and life-affirming experiences. Their conscience would get in the way. Your conscience is not your conscious mind, and it is something deeper and more fundamental which no one can override.

Will I Do Something Weird or Embarrassing While Under Hypnosis?

You are in the driver's seat. So, your behavior will remain under your control. Many people are seen doing funny or weird things in stage shows, where the hypnotist asks them to act something out, barking like a dog, for instance. This is for the sake of entertainment, and the participant will go along with it as part of a social contract of being in the hypnosis show. They are playing the role, not because they have no will, but because they want to! They went to the show, and they got up on stage willingly, and they are playing along.

Is hypnosis sleep?

No. Hypnosis is not sleeping. You remain aware and awake. The body is very relaxed, and the eyes are closed, so the person who is under hypnosis may look like they are sleeping, but they are not.

Is Hypnosis Psychotherapy?

It is not. Hypnosis is distinct from therapy in that way. Psychotherapists and other therapists may use hypnosis as a tool in their practice, but it is not one and the same.

Do I Need A License To Practice Hypnosis?

The requirements vary depending on where you live. In some countries, there are no laws regulating hypnosis. In others, you are required to take certified training and complete a minimum number of practice hours, as well as register to be a hypnotist. In Australia, there are no regulations, and in the United States, the regulations vary from state to state. It's the same in Europe from country to country. Research your area online to find out what is required in your particular situation.

What Are My Responsibilities As A Hypnotist?

You are taking someone on and helping them, and it's important to take this seriously and consider them. Hypnosis is intended to assist them in reaching their goals. So it's really all about them, and you are offering a tool to reach that goal. As such, they must be treated kindly. Be honest about your training, your level of experience, and the ability to help. Inform them about the process of hypnosis, what it does and doesn't do. Fill them in on what the process will be like and what they can expect from working with you.

What Is Hypnosis Not For?

Hypnosis cannot treat everything. A qualified physician must address certain physical problems and health problems. People who are suffering from serious mental illness, are deeply depressed, or are drug addicts are advised to seek specialized care.

Does Hypnosis Always Work?

The effectiveness of hypnosis depends on the person seeking help as well as the practitioner. The higher the skill level of the practitioner, the more likely they will be able to incite change, but the person must want to change, and that degree of motivation and will vary from person to person. The degree to which the habit is engrained also plays a role. Very strong addictions like smoking are more challenging or take more time.

Is Hypnosis the Same As Doing Positive Affirmations?

Hypnosis may use affirmations, and it does offer positive suggestions, but it is not the same as doing positive affirmations. The process of making the body and the mind relax is a skill used by a hypnotist to move your conscious mind out of the way and make the suggestions much more potent. The hypnotist has the ability to speak directly with the subconscious mind. This often makes it much more effective and quicker than repeating positive affirmations without any of the other processes.

Can Animals Be Hypnotized?

Debates about this are present; however, when you contemplate what hypnosis is, the process of accessing the subconscious mind with the goal of self-improvement, the answer is no. Animals cannot be hypnotized. Rather, what we see, or what looks like hypnosis with animals, is their ability to understand given commands as a result of training. The animal may go into what looks like sleep, but that doesn't mean we are speaking to its unconscious mind. It is responding very simply and obediently to certain body language that a trained person has skillfully perfected.

Hopefully, this covers the majority of questions and concerns and misconceptions about hypnosis, to give you a full and informed understanding of what it does and doesn't do, and the ins and outs of the profession as a business.

Chapter 5. What is Self-Hypnosis?

Self-hypnosis is a powerful method in which you talk right the subconscious mind or part of your brain. It gives you a way to eliminate any obstacles and confusion within the dialogue of your mind-body.

Self-hypnosis is still considered a mystical phenomenon by many people, even though this technique can be seen as prayer. You are alone, and you concentrate on your well-being. If you like, you ask God or a supreme being you believe in to help you. This practice also includes meditation (just like praying does), as well as chanting, mantras, inner confirmation or affirmation. When you have to perform at work or college, you make such statements like "I don't fear; I'm fine"; "I can do it" or exactly the opposite, like "I can't do it. Everybody is better than me," etc. Even when we imagine ourselves in a different scenario from what is currently happening, we are programming ourselves. What you are doing is continuously hypnotizing yourself. Self-hypnosis helps us to come into contact with the unconscious through the use of a specific language, aimed at awakening some parts of ourselves by leveraging archetypal symbols. Self-hypnotization is self-programming. Our unconscious understands the symbolic messages of words rather than their rational meaning; that's why figurative language is used in hypnosis for inducing the individual to relax and to focus on the inner world. We are embedding a vivid, information-rich image with emotions in the subconscious mind.

However, we must learn to pray, or let's say hypnotize ourselves accurately! Self-hypnosis is the_ability to apply techniques and procedures alone to stimulate the unconscious to become our ally and involve it directly in the realization of our goals. By learning the essential elements of communication with the unconscious mind, it is possible to become able to reprogram activities of our unconscious. Self-hypnosis is a method that does not dismiss the support of a professional but has the advantage of being able to be performed independently. This is possible through the use of CDs and DIY courses made by hypnotists to make this practice accessible to a larger number of people with significant advantages, even from an economic point of view!

It is merely a process of moving variables; you become the inductee of the relaxed state and the one who suggests the positive ideas for change on yourself. You are both the guide into the relaxed state and the one experiencing the relaxed state. While this might seem like it ups the ante and makes the process much more complicated just by increasing your number of roles and responsibilities, it is much simpler than you could ever imagine.

What is Self-Hypnosis For?

It was Milton H. Erickson, founder of modern hypnotherapy, who gave an exhaustive illustration of the effects and purposes of hypnosis and self-hypnosis. The scholar stated that this practice aims to communicate with the subconscious of the subjects through the use of metaphors and stories full of symbolic meanings (Tyrrell, 2014).

If incorrectly applied, self-hypnosis can certainly not harm, but it may not be useful in attaining the desired results, with the risk of not feeling motivated to continue a constructive relationship with the unconscious.

However, to do it as efficiently as possible, we need to be in a relaxed state of mind. So, accordingly, we start with relaxation to gather the attention inside, while suspending conscious control. Then we insert suggestions and affirmations to the unconscious mind. At the end of the time allocated for the process, a gradual awakening procedure facilitates the return to the state of permanent consciousness. When you are calm, your subconscious is 20-25% more programmable than when you are agitated. Also, it effectively relieves stress (you can repair a lot of information and stimuli you understand), aids regeneration, energizes, triggers positive physiological changes, improves concentration, helps you find solutions, and helps you make the right decisions. If the state of conscious trance is reached, then if the patient manages to let himself go by concentrating on the words of the hypnotist, progressively forgetting the external stimuli, the physiological parameters undergo considerable variations. The confirmation comes from science, and in fact, it was found that during hypnosis, the left hemisphere, the rational one, decreases its activity in favor of the more creative hemisphere, the right one (Harris, n. d.).

You can do self-hypnosis in faster and more immediate ways, even during the course of the various daily activities after you have experienced what state you need to reach during hypnosis.

A better understanding of communication with the unconscious mind highlights how indispensable our collaboration is to slip into the state outside the ordinary consciousness. In other words, we enter an altered state of consciousness because we want it, and every form of hypnosis, even if induced by someone else, is always self-hypnosis.

We wish to access the extraordinary power of unconscious creativity; for this, we understand that it is necessary to put aside for a while the control of the rational mind and let ourselves slip entirely into relaxation and into the magical world of the unconscious where everything is possible. Immense benefits can be obtained from a relationship that becomes natural and habitual with one's own unconscious. Self-hypnosis favors the emergence of constructive responses from our being, can allow us to know ourselves better, helps us to be more aware of our potential, and more able to express them and use them to foster our success in every field of possible application.

Chapter 6. A Step by Step Guide To Self-Hypnotization

There are several self-hypnosis techniques out there; however, they are all based on one concept: focusing on a single idea, object, image, or word. This is the key that will be opening the door to trance. You can achieve focus in many ways, which is the reason why there are so many different techniques that can be applied. After a period of initial learning, those who have learned a method, and have continued to practice it, realize that they can skip certain steps. In this part, we will take a look at the essential self-hypnosis techniques.

Relaxation is key here, and the pathways to it are many and numbered. What relaxes you? It can be listening to music, reading a book, or watching television. When you do any of these things, your conscious mind is being "hypnotized" by your own actions. The song, the book, the film—these are the pendulums we are swinging in front of our own eyes. And what is being suggested to us by them? The things our mind consumes every day are post-hypnotic suggestions we are feeding to our sub-conscious mind. We must become aware of them. If the song you are listening to says, "I want to die. I am sick of this world," you will come to want to die and be sick of this world. If the film or television program you are watching is negative, you will become negativistic. If the book you are reading promotes hate-speech, you will come to be a hateful person. It is the very nature of learning—what we focus on is what grows in our psyche. We must thoroughly understand the power of focus and intention, will, and willpower. We must meditate on where our focus is going in our daily living and make the decisions to focus on more positive areas of infinite being. This goes beyond outside influences such as media and other people we interact with all the way up to the most important influential factor on our wellbeing, our thoughts and feelings, our beliefs, that being ourselves.

Self-hypnotism will be you, in reality, finding a safe place, sitting down, breathing in and out in peace, and heading inside—heading inside your brain, or your heart, or your soul, heading inside of your consciousness. See who you are, who you view yourself as, what you think, what you do, then tell yourself who you are going to be. Tell yourself what you are going to assume from here on out. How you are going to feel about yourself going forward. "I am healthy. I am wellness. I am my own master. No one controls me. I control my destiny. I am the decider of my actions. I am not indebted to anyone or anything. I am free. I am great. I will be the best that I can be."

Find your mantras. What do you desire? Do you want peace? Your mantra can be, "I will be at peace." Relax, take several deep breaths, envision yourself floating on a cloud, in the hands of a powerful deity, like the Hindus, or at the core of the brightest star in the universe, having it emanates from you, and say, over and over, louder and louder, firmer and firmer, "I am peace." You are what you desire. Hone your desires. Understand where your focus and intentions are. Self-hypnotism is something that is practiced by every single person every single day. It is unconscious. Our subconscious minds have a void that needs to be filled by intention; it is a continually running program consuming information.

Find your inner peace. Find your temple. Find your mantra. Examine yourself from an outside perspective and find out who you really want to be, what you would like to see looking in the mirror, and what you would believe to be your absolute, ultimate peak. We will erase the pathways in our mind that lead us to stumble blindly into the negative spaces we know so well and carve out new pathways that lead us into brand new positive paradises that we can only imagine. And we will do it, quite simply, by the very act of imagining them itself. The power of our thoughts cannot be overstated. You are what you think you are. You are not what anyone else thinks you are. You are not what you are. You are whatever you want to be.

There are a few guidelines to hypnosis, and they guarantee that your training is the most proficient and yields the best advantages. At the point when you are prepared to start utilizing the sound, locate an agreeable and safe spot in your home or office where you can sit in a seat, lean back, or even rests. Ensure you are loose and in a spot where you don't need to focus on whatever else. Try not to tune in to your daze work while you are driving a vehicle or working any kind of hardware. It is useful to settle on a customary time every day or night to rehearse your self-hypnosis. Sleep time is a decent chance to make the most of your stupor work, and rehearsing as of now can be a great method to enter a tranquil sleep.

Interruptions and interferences are unavoidable. As opposed to permitting them to bother you and remove you from your stupor work, use them. Utilize the sounds in the earth around you to improve your daze understanding. For instance, while doing your hypnosis, you may see a sound and begin imagining that this sound is diverting you. You, at that point, become more centered on this interruption than on your hypnosis. You might be enticed to battle against it—which removes vitality from the hypnosis. Rather, when you notice a sound that from the outset appears diverting or irritating, assume responsibility for it by giving it your authorization to be there as a foundation sound. Give it a task, for example, contemplating internally that "the sound of the yapping hound is helping me go deeper and deeper inside" or "the fan engine seems like a cascade that is an alleviating foundation sound." At our private practice in Tucson, there is a day school that unavoidably lets the youngsters out to play during one of our hypnosis meetings. That is the point at which we recommend, "The sound of youngsters can be a foundation sound that releases you deeper and deeper inside yourself now." This is a piece of our "utilization everything" theory.

Interruptions additionally incorporate the sensations you may understanding inside you. For instance, you may end up seeing a piece of your body that tingles. The more you center around the tingling or on scratching the tingle, the less you are concentrating your awareness on the daze. On those occasions, you remind yourself that you have consent to move your consideration back to your daze or dream and let the tingle go unscratched. When working with patients who have torment issue, we instruct them to center consideration away from the "interruption" of torment along these lines. All things considered, we can't control the earth around us or the sensations inside us; however, we can pick where we concentrate. If you experience difficulty relinquishing an irritating interruption, you may need to order that it be there as a foundation

—

37

sound or sensation, which at that point releases you all the more serenely inside. Withdraw yourself from anything that is contending with your thoughtfulness regarding your hypnosis. Relinquish any battle with nature. Simply let it be there, and sometime you will receive no longer notification it. At the point when you figure out how to acknowledge a sensation, clamor, or another component that meddles with your hypnosis, you no longer permit it to have authority over you.

Law of Reversed Effect

There is a law in hypnosis, called the Law of Reversed Effect, that says that occasionally the more you attempt to accomplish something, the more it doesn't occur. A model is a point at which you need to state a name that you realize, you know—it might be a book title, an individual, a film—however, you can't state it at that point, and the more you attempt, the less it is there. The name comes when you propose to your subconscious mind that "I'll recollect later" or "It'll come to me later." By relinquishing the inquiry, "What's the name? What's the name?" you have discharged your subconscious mind to now recover and convey the appropriate response, and it generally does. Along these lines, the Law of Reversed Effect is that when you are making a decent attempt for something, it just gives you the inverse (the opposite).

Stages of Self-Hypnosis

Getting ingested in your considerations and thoughts is that delicate excursion into the focal point of yourself called "going into a stupor." The straightforward methods of self-hypnosis incorporate going into a daze, deepening the daze, utilizing that daze state to give messages and recommendations to the mind-body, and coming out of the daze.

38

Subconscious Mind (Or Unconscious Mind)

This is the bit of our mind that performs capacities and procedures beneath our reasoning mindfulness. It is the mind of the body. It inhales us, digests, beats our hearts, and as a rule, deals with our automatic physical procedures for us. It can likewise instruct us to pick a bit of new mango rather than chocolate cake, to quit eating when we are full, or to appreciate a stroll in the recreation center.

Going into Trance

When you are utilizing the stupor at this point, take a shot at the sound, I will be your guide as you go into a daze. I will utilize a daze enlistment strategy that you will discover quieting and centering. You have most likely observed the swinging watch technique in motion pictures, which is thirty-five years of training I have never observed anybody use. Yet, there is a vast kind of approaches to concentrate on going into a stupor. You may gaze at a spot on the divider, utilize a breathing procedure, or utilize dynamic body unwinding. You will hear an assortment of acceptance strategies on the stupor work sound. They are just the prompts or the signs that you are providing for yourself to state, "I am going into a daze" or "I will do my hypnosis currently." Going into stupor can likewise be thought of as "letting yourself dream ... intentionally." You are letting yourself become consumed in your contemplations and thoughts, exceptionally ingested, and permitting yourself to imagine or envision what you want as accomplished and genuine. There is no "going under." Instead, there is a beautiful encounter of going inside.

Cognizant Mind

This is the "thinking mind" or the piece of the mind that gives us our mindfulness or feeling of knowing and oversees our deliberate capacities. For instance, our cognizant mind takes that second bit of pie at the meal, swipes the check card at the market, and moves the fork to our mouth.

Chapter 7. Different Methods of Self-Hypnosis

The Betty Erickson Method

Here I'll summarize the most practical points of this method of Betty Erickson, wife of Milton Erickson, the most famous hypnotist of 1900. Choose something you don't like about yourself. Turn it into an image, and then turn this image into a positive one. If you don't like your body shape, take a picture of your body, then turn it into an image of your beautiful self with a body you would like to have. Before inducing self-hypnosis, give yourself a time limit before hypnotizing yourself mentally or better yet, saying aloud the following sentence, "I induce self-hypnosis for X minutes." Your mind will take time like a Swiss watch.

How do you practice?

Take three objects around you, preferably small and bright, like a door handle, a light spot on a painting, etc. and fix your attention on each one of them. Take three sounds from your environment, traffic, fridge noise, etc., and fix your attention on each one. Take three sensations you are feeling, the itchy nose, tingling in the leg, the feeling of air passing through the nose, etc. It's better to use unusual sensations, to which attention is not usually drawn, such as the sensation of the right foot inside the shoe. Don't fix your attention for too long, just enough to make you aware of what you are seeing, feeling, or trying. The mind is quick. Then, in the same way, switch to two objects, two sounds, two sensations. Always be calm, while switching to an object, a sound, a sensation. If you have perfectly done things, you are in a trance, ready for the next step.

Now let your mind wander, as you did in class when the teacher spoke and you looked out of the window, and you were in another place, in another time, in another space, in a place where you would have liked to be, so completely forget about everything else. Now recall the initial image. Perhaps the mind wanders, from time to time it gets distracted, maybe it goes adrift, but it doesn't matter. As soon as you can, take the initial image, and start working on it. Do not make efforts to try to remind you of what it means or what it is. Your mind works according to mental associations, let it work at its best without unnecessarily disturbing it: it knows what it must do. Manipulate the image, play with it a little. See if it looks brighter, or if it is smaller, or it is more pleasant. If it is a moving image, send it back and forth in slow motion or speed it up. When the initial image always gets worse, replace it instantly with the second image.

Reorientation, also known as awakening, marks the end of self-hypnotic induction. Enjoy your new image, savor it as much as you like, and when you have done this, open your eyes. If you are unable to give yourself enough time, limits before entering self-hypnosis, when you are satisfied with the work done, count quietly to yourself from one to ten and wake up, and open your eyes (Traversa, 2018).

The Benson Method

Herbert Benson, in his famous book titled, Relaxation Response, describes the methods and results of some tests carried out on a group of meditators dedicated to "transcendental meditation" to reach concentration (1975). Benson suggested a method of relaxation based on the concentration of the mind on a single idea, which was incorporated in the Eastern disciplines. The technique includes the following steps:

- Meditate on one word, but you can choose an object or something else if you want to.

- Now, its time sitting down in a quiet place and close your eyes. Relax the muscles and direct attention to the breath.

- Think silently about the object of meditation and continue to do so for 10-20 minutes. If you find that you have lost the object of meditation, gather your focus again on the original object.

- Once the set time is reached, open your eyes stretch yourself well for some additional minutes. Obviously, to perform better, you will need to practice.

Benson proposes this exercise as a meditation practice. In reality, there are no differences between the hypnotic state and that achieved with meditation. This is one of the most straightforward self-hypnosis exercises you can do.

Here is another simple technique that was developed by the first hypnotists because it leads to a satisfactory state of trance in a reasonable time. It can be used to enter self-hypnosis in a short time.

- Now, its time sitting down in a quiet place and close your eyes Relax the muscles and direct attention to the breath.

- Begin to open and close your eyes by counting slowly. Open your eyes at the odd numbers close them at the even numbers. Continue counting very slowly and slowing down the numbering of even numbers.

- After a few numbers, your eyes become tired, and you find it difficult to open them at odd numbers. Continue counting while you can open your eyes at the odd numbers. If you cannot do it, it means you are in a trance.

- Go deeper by slowly counting twenty other numbers. Let yourself go to the images, to the sensations, and to the words that come to mind. To wake up from the trance, count from one to five, and open your eyes at five (Stress Management Plus, n. d.).

These are examples of techniques, but no one is preventing you from devising others, as long as the underlying assumption is maintained: concentration on a single idea.

We, as a whole, essentially need time to unwind, to dream, to imagine. It is refreshing to the physical body and restoring to the soul. At the point when we practice our hypnosis, it offers us simply that: an exceptionally close to home time to animate and enhance our mind and body. The training is done essentially. You don't require anything over an agreeable and safe spot.

Chapter 8. How to Enhance Self-Hypnosis Experience

Know If Your Self Hypnosis Is Working

There are some small things you can do physically to know if hypnosis is really working for you, especially if you are a self-hypnosis beginner.

Put both your hands together, palm-to-palm tightly and keep them in this position throughout your hypnotic state. Imagine your hands superglued together and keep saying, "my hands can't come apart. They are stuck together". Now try to pull them apart. If you are not able to do so, then you're in the right state of hypnosis.

Another method to test the effectiveness of your self-hypnosis is to concentrate on how heavy one of your arms is becoming and if it is getting heavier and heavier throughout your session. Imagine a heavyweight is placed on your arm, which is making it difficult to lift your arm. Now try to raise that arm up into the air. If you are failing at doing this, then you are in the right hypnosis state.

What to Do If Self Hypnosis Doesn't Work

Have you ever encountered the annoyance of having a name on your tongue tip? The more you try to recall the name, the more difficult it gets to remember. And then, when you relax, the name automatically comes back to you.

At times, we prevent ourselves from achieving our goals when we try too hard. The approach you make towards self-hypnosis will determine how quickly and easily you get a grasp of it. Avoid trying too hard or setting unrealistic goals. Relax and take your time. Welcome the pace at which you obtain results, regardless of how small they may at first appear. Trust yourself, and you'll go on to obtain the success you want.

Mistakes That Often People Make

Learning self-hypnosis is not that hard, but it is easy for newbies to make mistakes. However, try to avoid making the following beginners mistakes when you begin learning self-hypnosis, and you'll be off to a great start:

- Expecting Too Much

Many people regard self-hypnosis as a miracle cure and thus become disappointed if they don't get the desired result in their very first attempt. Never expect to achieve your goal with just one or two sessions, especially if you are a newbie. You need to allow it to take time in order to be effective.

- Failure to Relax Enough

You are required to quiet your body and mind to maintain a hypnotic state. Regular meditation will assist you in learning the focus that you will need in order to utilize self-hypnosis effectively.

- Failure of Being Open to the Self Hypnosis Experience

You'll need to work through any psychological blocks you have about hypnosis before doing a hypnotic session.

- Failure to Prepare Enough Ahead of Time

Hypnotherapy takes time and preparation to use it as an effective therapeutic tool. Keep in mind that, like any other skill, self-hypnosis needs to be learned and practiced before you can perform it well and obtain your desired benefits.

Tips to Manifest Your Best Through Self Hypnosis

- Keep Yourself Hydrated

Drink water before the session to ensure that you are hydrated since being hydrated is helpful in any practice of negative energy clearing.

- Be Relaxed

Relaxation is an important element of self-hypnosis since when you relax the mind and body, then this is when you clear the way of an opportunity to welcome effective life changing changes. Through self-hypnosis is constructed to provide you relaxation, you can further enhance the experience by getting rid of your tension and stress by having a home massage or a relaxation bath, or doing some form of exercise.

- Avoid Struggling with Your Emotions

As a newbie, it can be frustrating and difficult to obtain a peaceful mind state. Clearing your mind may induce the flow of different kinds of emotions and make you unstable. Try to overlook these emotions and concentrate more on finding peace in your mind.

Last and an essential thing you must know is to enhance your hypnotic experience is that it's ok if you're unable to achieve. The world won't come to a standstill, the sun won't stop rising; neither will the sky come falling if you're not able to obtain your goals. Success and failure both are cyclic in nature and are a part of our life.

Thus, don't get obsessed with goals, rather be passionate about it. Work towards it never ends up spending more time worrying about it. Sooner or later, you'll surely be the winner.

Chapter 9. Weight Loss With Mini Habits

Mindfulness and Mindful Eating

The best time to introduce mindfulness is immediately after your meditation. This is a period when you have stopped meditating, but you are not yet ready to go back into the hustle-bustle of life. Mindfulness involves thinking about the moment that you are in. This means that there is no room for thoughts of the past and certainly no room for worries about the future. After your meditation is over and your journal is complete, sit with your eyes open and learn to be in the moment by observing everything around you. That may be something that you see within the flicker of a candle. It may be feeling the ambiance of the room, or it may be taking in the aroma of the room. Think of nothing except for those things that your senses pick up on. If you find your mind wandering, bring yourself back to focus on this moment.

We are all told what's right and what's wrong and, much of the time, develop hang-ups about how we are to behave. That's perfectly normal in any society. However, what we do tend to worry about is how we conform to the ideas and ideals of society. Are you too fat? Are you too thin? Are you tall enough? Are you pretty enough? All of these things feed our self-esteem to the extent that most people will look into a mirror and not be one hundred percent happy about what they see. Mindfulness in observation will help. The idea is that you observe people and, in doing so, dismiss all of the judgment aspects. Sit in a crowded place and just watch people. Be aware of the way that their bodies move. Be aware of the laughter of children. This moment offers you so many valuable experiences, but what the Buddhist philosophy includes is something

48

that is called "rightful seeing." That means that you observe without any form of judgment whatsoever. You simply see yourself as an outsider observing, rather than a critic.

What this kind of observation does is teach you acceptance. It makes you more capable of being empathetic. It allows you to place yourself into other people's shoes, and that's a very valuable thing indeed. Look at facial expressions. Take in the way people are behaving and also the way that they are interacting with each other, but remember to take the judgment element out of the picture. If you are mindful of others, you are much more likely to interact with them in a positive manner. It also helps you to see beyond the obvious and see the world with compassion. That's a very valuable thing to feel and makes you more of a person than you would otherwise be.

Mindfulness is simply what it says on the label. It is mindful. It is taking note of what is happening when it happens and learning from it. To practice mindfulness, look at the way that you think. When you find that your mind is wandering to another time, you need to appreciate that if you are living the now within another time, you lose the opportunity of making NOW count for anything. Yesterday has gone. Tomorrow has not yet arrived. Practice living in the now. It may be all that you have.

Mindfulness Exercise

In this mindfulness exercise, we need you to find somewhere inspirational. Whatever gives you the wow factor will be a suitable place. This can be a garden, a beauty spot, or somewhere that you find peace and calm, such as a beach at sunrise or sunset or even standing on top of a hill. The reason we need you to be in this kind of environment is that the exercise is one in humility. Humility is what you feel when you know that the world around you are bigger than you are. The beauty of a flower will show you that, just as the golden color of a leaf in autumn will. Be inspired by what you see and keep all other thoughts out of your mind. You need to see how small you are in comparison with this beauty because sometimes we forget that. This smallness may seem to be a negative aspect of your life, but it really isn't. It puts things into perspective in a very positive way. Although you are small, you are one of the wonders that nature has produced. Thus, you are every bit as important as all of the wonder you see around you.

Sit down somewhere comfortable, and if you wish to take a meditation stance, then this is acceptable. Now use your senses and banishing all other thoughts from your mind, take in the following aspects of what you are looking at:

- The colors
- The aromas
- The sounds
- The contrasts
- The calm

Reflecting on all of these things are always going to be beneficial, but if you are stressed, then choosing an inspirational place will help you to be mindful and to feel all of the beauty. Breathe as you do when you meditate, though be aware of everything around you and let the thoughts that go through your mind concentrate on your senses, rather than letting them stray into other times and other problems. Let go.

Chapter 10. The Importance of Making Mindful Eating a Habit

We eat mindlessly. The principal explanation behind our awkwardness with nourishment and eating is that we have overlooked how to be available as we eat. Careful eating is the act of developing a receptive familiarity with how the nourishment we eat influences one's body, sentiments, brain, and all that is around us. The training improves our comprehension of what to eat, how to eat, the amount to eat, and why we eat what we eat. When eating carefully, we are completely present and relish each chomp - connecting every one of our faculties to really value the nourishment. Past simple tastes, we see the appearance, sounds, scents, and surfaces of our nourishment, just as our mind's reaction to these perceptions.

The precepts of care apply to careful eating, too; however, the idea of careful eating goes past the person. It likewise incorporates how what you eat influences the world. When we eat with this comprehension and understanding, appreciation and empathy will emerge inside us. Accordingly, careful eating is fundamental to guarantee nourishment supportability for who and what is to come, as we are persuaded to pick nourishments that are useful for our wellbeing, yet in addition useful for our planet.

It is outstanding that most get-healthy plans do not work in the long haul. Around 85% of individuals with heftiness who shed pounds come back to or surpass their underlying load inside a couple of years. Binge eating, passionate eating, outside seating, and eating because of nourishment longings have been connected to weight put on, and weight recovers after effective weight reduction. Interminable presentation to stress may likewise assume an enormous job in gorging and heftiness. By changing the manner in which you consider nourishment, the negative sentiments that might be related to eating are supplanted with mindfulness, improved poise, and positive feelings. At the point when undesirable eating practices are tended to, your odds of long-haul weight reduction achievement are expanded.

When you are eating, make sure you are taking some time to absorb the experience of your meal truly. Chew slowly, really notice each flavor in your meal, and take your time in between bites. When you feel satisfied, do not force yourself to eat more. Do not rush yourself, and do not treat it as a chore. Instead, truly experience the process. You will likely learn a lot about yourself and your preferences during this process.

Often, we treat eating like a chore. We go to drive-thru restaurants, or we eat convenience meals, and we leave out the experience of cooking and preparing our meal. We don't get the experience of plating it and truly looking at it before we eat it because we are in such a rush to eat it as quickly as possible and resume our busy lifestyles. Instead of doing this, make the entire process a mindfulness practice. Take your time when you are preparing the meal, plate it carefully in a way that looks attractive to you, and take your time eating it. Your health will improve significantly as well, as you will not be overeating or indulging in unhealthy food choices anymore.

Food is such an essential part of our lives, yet we treat it with very little care. The preparation and consumption of food are often treated as a chore, and we very rarely think about food as fuel for our bodies.

Mindful eating starts right from the moment you go grocery shopping. I do mean grocery shopping, as in buying raw ingredients and then cooking them into meals. I do not mean visiting your nearest fast food restaurant or searching for something that can be microwaved into something barely edible.

Chemical additives and processed foods and have ruined our palettes to the extent that we do not even taste real food anymore. When you first switch to a whole food diet, you'll notice that you won't be able to taste a lot of the food you eat. This is because the flavors present in processed food are raised to an unhealthy degree, and these foods are full of sugar. The net result is that your taste buds have been dulled and they need stimulation in order to figure out what it is you're eating.

When shopping, take your time to look at the different colors of food available. Marvel at the differences in texture, size, and shapes of each ingredient. I'm not advocating converting to veganism or anything of the sort. Ultimately, everything we eat is food, and this includes animals as well. Whether this is OK with you or not is up to your beliefs. Your aim should be to eat as balanced a diet as possible, and this means including food from different food groups and blending as many colors into your food as possible.

This is a neat trick to figure out how balanced your diet is actually. The more varied the texture and colors in your food, the better the odds are that you're hitting your nutritional needs. Isn't it marvelous how nature has given us this easy way of determining this without needing to walk around with a calculator all the time?

As you prepare your food, infuse it with love and wish for it to provide nutrition and life to all those who consume it. When cooking, notice how the texture of the food changes and how all these diverse ingredients come together under heat to form a single dish. I'm not trying to get you to become a chef here, but the way raw ingredients come together to form a whole really is a miraculous process.

Where is your mind when you're eating your food usually? Probably on the TV or distracted with something else. Mealtimes are treated as a chore in most households, and this really is a shame. Even if the whole family comes together for a meal, the objective isn't to enjoy the food; it is to talk about our day and to settle any lingering issues.

Take the time to notice what your food really tastes like and how it feels in your mouth. Acknowledge that this food is going inside you to fuel you and is a key contributor to your health. In modern society, we have a truly terrible relationship with food. Thanks to the rise of social media, our diets are under intense scrutiny, and lots of food groups are demonized.

Some eat only carbs, and some eat only fat. Some claim juicing is the best, and there's something called the fruit-based diet as well. Understand that all food is food. It doesn't matter what you eat as long as it is naturally sourced as possible and that you eat it in the right quantities. Even junk food has its place, since eating the occasional burger will help you feel better.

Ultimately, this is what food is supposed to do. Make you feel good about living. Seek to achieve a state of balance with your food, and it will return the favor to you via good health.

Mindful eating, on its own, is not a diet. It does not have any kind of juice cleanses, and neither does it require you to eliminate any kinds of food. It also does not tell you when to eat, and there are no promises of quick fixes. Mindful eating is more a framework or guide that helps you eat better and make better choices with your food. It puts you as the decision-maker of all your choices, so you choose what to eat to meet your fitness and weight goals. Through mindful eating, you are not eating just as a means to an end. It is not about choosing foods based on our desired outcome. This is potentially self-defeating. All mindful eating does is to invite ourselves to be present while we cook, and eat our foods, to savor without any guilt or judgment, anxiety, or inner commentary.

This method is all about spending less time focused on what your weight would be or should be and all kinds of storylines about your weight and instead, embracing eating in a way that helps people find the weight that is right for them. Conventional dieting and eating plans would cause too much stress around eating, even if the plan wasn't meant for it to be like that. Still, because we put in heaps of pressure and intensity together with false expectations, most of the time, we end up ruining our diet and eating plans.

Through mindful eating, we want to eliminate the view of food being a reward or punishment. Because we view food like this, we end up saying we 'deserve' a huge slice of chocolate cake because we view it as a treat after going through 24 hours of fasting or going one week on a celery juice diet or even eating less than 500 calories for an entire month. People who want to lose weight are obsessed with wanting to be thin that we either end up undereating or suppressing our feelings of hunger, or we just end up ignoring our signs of being full.

The mind is calmer when we are more aware, and when the mind is calm, we are less agitated or stressed, and the less we eat emotionally. When we are more focused, we also increase our clarity to look at the choices we make on food and make better attempts to eat better food choices. When we are calmer and clearer, we are more content, more compassionate on our weight, and ourselves, and we also become more aware that sustainable weight loss is a journey.

Mindful eating is about bringing mindfulness back to the dining table, and this also means a kinder and gentler approach towards eating. It is not about changing our diets but more about changing our relationship and thoughts about food.

You may think this is a strange topic, but when you look at the way that people live their lives these days, you will know that there is nothing strange about it. People rush to eat their food. They don't allow their bodies to actually enjoy the taste and texture of what they eat. In fact, some will eat breakfast on the move because they haven't allowed themselves time to do it. Not only is this bad for your body, but it's not doing your equilibrium much good either. The next time that you want to eat, makes sure that you have time to sit down and enjoy it. If this means leaving the office at lunchtime and going out to the park with your sandwich, then do it.

As you taste your food, be aware of what you are eating. Enjoy the tastes and the textures. Chew your food correctly and take your time with your eating. Be totally in the moment, and enjoy the warmth or cool feel of food on your tongue. Enjoy the crackle of food. Enjoy the burst of taste on your tongue. Mindfulness encompasses the moment and does not go beyond it. Thus, when you are eating, think only of the eating and start to feel your senses opening to the delight of the experience. Smell the aromas and feel that cup of warm coffee sensually working its way around your mouth and warming you.

Chapter 11. The Power Of Mindset

When it comes to making any sort of change in life, the approach you take will make or break your success. If you choose an approach that doesn't work well with your specific personality, the likelihood of relapse occurring will be extremely high.

Taking an approach that is focused on perfection leaves you feeling down on yourself and like a failure most of the time. Because this causes you to notice that you are not perfect instead of focusing on the good parts, the progress you have made will always make you feel like you are not doing enough or that you have not made enough progress. Since you will never achieve perfection as this is impossible for anyone, you will never feel satisfaction or allow yourself to celebrate your achievements. You must recognize that this will be something complicated, but that you will do it anyways. If you force yourself into change like a drill sergeant and with an aggressive mindset, you will end up beating yourself up every day for something. Forcing yourself will not lead to a long-lasting change, as you will eventually become fed up with all of the rules you have placed on yourself, and you will just want to abandon the entire mission. If you approach the change with rigidity, you will not allow yourself time to look back on your achievements and celebrate yourself, to have a tasty meal that is good for your soul every once in a while, and you may fall off of your plan in a more extreme way than you were before. You may end up having a week-long binge and falling into worse habits than you had before.

Your mindset plays a huge role in your success when it comes to change. The way that you view your journey will make or break it and will determine whether or not your change is lasting or fleeting, and whether or not you really become invested in making the changes in your life. While you need to push yourself to do anything hard, the key is knowing when to ease up on yourself a little bit and when to push harder. Recognizing and responding to this is much more effective than putting your nose to the grindstone every day and becoming burnt out, tired, and left without any more willpower. To continue on the long and challenging journey that a lifestyle change involves, you must give yourself a break now and then. Think of this like running a marathon, where you will need to go about it slowly and purposefully with a strategy in mind. If you ran into a marathon full-speed and refused to slow down or look back at all, you would lose energy, stamina, and motivation in quite a short amount of time and turn back or run off the side of the road feeling defeated and as if you failed. Looking at this example, you can see that this person did not fail. They just approached the marathon with the wrong strategy and that they would have been completely capable of finishing that marathon if they had taken their time, followed a plan, and slowed down every once in a while to regain their strength. Even if they walked the marathon slowly for hours and hours, eventually, they would make it over that finish line. They would probably also do so feeling proud, accomplished, and like a new person. This is how we want to view this journey or any journey of self-improvement. Even if you are able to do only one tiny step each day, you are making a step toward your goal, and that is the important part.

The Power of Imagination

The way to harness your suggestibility is to know what \ to say to yourself and how to say it. Talking yourself, thin j can be done without actually uttering an audible word. / People talk to themselves all the time. In some rare cases A they startle you by talking out loud. Even those who \ mumble or move their lips are stand-outs enough to make me you wonder. Most of us talk to ourselves silently, with (thoughts that are either in word form or image form. In either case, it is our imagination that is utilized. The power of the imagination is the greatest power on earth. Every accomplishment in this material world has first been imagined. It is the step before the written word, design, or blueprint. There is even evidence that what we do not want, but hold in the imagination through fear, comes. In the body, imagination sets off stimuli. Imagine a sizzling steak, and the saliva begins to flow. You could not set off your saliva by sheer willpower, no matter how hard you tried. It is imagination that causes impotence, fear of water, and a multitude of emotional disorders.

Harnessed to motivate in a positive direction, imagination can work miracles in health and well-being. Talking to yourself is an exercise in imagining. You put your imagination through the proper paces, and then you learn how to develop it and train it. You permit it to work closely with your subconscious, unobstructed by your conscious thoughts. As a team, they are unconquerable. Look at the uselessness of willpower in drug addiction, gambling, alcoholism. You have your own experience to prove the uselessness of willpower in weight control. To abandon useless willpower and to embrace useful imagination power is to ensure permanent success in self- mastery.

Chapter 12. Strategies for the Mind

Easing into a lifestyle change is the best way to go about something like this because of the way that our minds work. We don't like looking forward to our lives and feeling like we will have no control over what we are going to do with it. By choosing smaller sections to break it up into, we can be more present in each moment, which makes making healthy choices easier. By doing so, all of these small sections add up to weeks, months, and eventually years of healthy options. Eventually, we have gone a year without turning to sweets in a moment of sadness and only chosen them when we are consciously choosing to treat ourselves. Another strategy that we can use for our minds is to reward yourself at milestones along your journey. At one week you can reward yourself with a date night at a restaurant, or at one month you can visit the new bakery down the street. This not only helps you to stay motivated because you are allowing yourself some of the joys you love, but it also keeps you motivated because you are allowing yourself to take time to look back at how far you have come and feel great about your progress. Allowing yourself to celebrate goes hand in hand with this, as well. When you make a good choice or plan what you will order at a restaurant before you get there, allowing yourself to feel happy and proud is very important. By doing this, you are showing yourself that you have done something great, that you are capable of making changes, and that you will allow yourself to feel good about these positive strides you have made instead of just looking to the next one all the time. If you were to ignore this and be of the mindset that nothing is good enough, you would end up feeling burnt out and quite down about the length of the process. Think of that marathon analogy again, and this is what can happen if we don't allow ourselves time to feel proud and accomplished for small victories along the way.

Another strategy for the mind is to avoid beating yourself up for falling off the wagon. This may happen sometimes. What we need to do, though, is to focus not on the fact that it has happened, but on how we are going to deal with and react to it. There are a variety of reactions that a person can have to this. We will examine the possible responses and the pros and cons below:

One is that they feel as though their progress is ruined and that they might as well begin another time again, so they go back to their old ways and may not try again for some time. This could happen many times over as they will fall off each time and then decide that they might as well give up this time and try again, but each time it ends the same.

Two, the person could fall off of their diet plan and tell themselves that this day is a write-off and that they will begin the next day again. The problem with this method is that continuing the rest of the day as you would have before you decided to make a change will make it so that the next day is like beginning all over again, and it will be very hard to start again. They may be able to begin the next day again, and it could be fine, but they must be able to motivate themselves if they are to do this. Knowing that you have fallen off before makes it so that you may feel down on yourself and feel as though you can't do it, so beginning again the next day is very important.

And they then decide that they will pick it up again the next week. This will be even harder than starting the next day again as multiple days of eating whatever you like will make it very hard to go back to making the healthy choices again afterward.

Four, after eating something that they wish they hadn't, and that wasn't a healthy choice, they will decide not to eat anything for the rest of the day so that they don't eat too many calories or too much sugar, and decide that the next day they will begin again. This is very difficult on the body as you are going to be quite hungry by the time bed rolls around. Instead of forgiving yourself, you are punishing yourself, and it will make it very hard not to reach for chips late at night when you are starving and feeling down.

Number five is what you should do in this situation. This option is the best for success and will make it the most likely that you will succeed long-term. If you fall off at lunch, let's say, because you are tired and, in a rush, and you just grab something from a fast-food restaurant instead of going home for lunch or buying something at the grocery store to eat, this is how we will deal with it. Firstly, you will likely feel like you have failed and may feel quite down about having made an unhealthy choice. Now instead of starving for the rest of the day or eating only lettuce for dinner, you will put this slip up at lunch behind you, and you will continue your day as if it never happened. You will eat a healthy dinner as you planned, and you will continue on with the plan. You will not wait until tomorrow to begin again, and you will continue as you would if you had made that healthy choice at lunch. The key to staying on track can bounce back. The people who can bounce back mentally are the ones who will be most likely to succeed. You will need to maintain a positive mental state and look forward to the rest of the day and the rest of the week in just the same way as you did before you had a slip-up. One unideal meal out of the entire week is not going to ruin all of your progress, and recovering from emotional eating is largely a mental game. It is more psychological than anything else, so we must not underestimate the role that our mindset plays in our success or failure.

How to Be Gentle with Yourself

It is important to be gentle with ourselves because we are usually our own toughest examiner. We look at ourselves very critically, and we often think that nothing we do is good enough. We must be gentle with ourselves so as not to discourage ourselves, put ourselves down, or make ourselves feel bad about what we are working so hard to accomplish. We must remind ourselves that everything in life is a process and does not happen instantly, and we mustn't tell ourselves to "hurry up and succeed," as we often do.

When you fall off track, you must not beat yourself up for this. It is essential to be gentle with yourself. When you beat yourself up, it will only cause you to turn into a spiral of negativity and continue to talk down to yourself. This will make you lose motivation and will make you feel like you are a failure. Having this state of mind will make it difficult not to turn to food for comfort. We must avoid this entire process by avoiding beating ourselves up in the first place. If we don't beat ourselves up and we instead encourage ourselves, instead of thinking of how we can't do it, and it is too hard and then needing to turn to food for comfort and a feeling of safety, we will not even make ourselves feel the need to find safety at all. Instead, we will talk to ourselves positively and encourage ourselves from within, which, instead of making ourselves feel bad, we will instead feel motivated, and we will be even more ready to continue on our journey.

Chapter 13. The Power Of Affirmations

Affirmations are powerful weight loss tools, and any other goal you want to accomplish in life. Affirmations are positive, short statements about something you want to attract or manifest written in the present tense. Asserting the word means "making it strong." The mind is like a machine. Affirmations work to help reprogram the subconscious mind like software programs.

Affirmations take advantage of your mind's power to create what you want. Affirmations aid you to have a focus on your intentions and help you stay on track. Using statements will make the goals for weight loss a reality.

Our affirmations are nothing more than repeated statements in a given situation, whereby we comment on the pleasant or unpleasant effects of that situation inside us. If you observe these inner comments, you will find that they are repetitive elements that we happen to say very often to ourselves. However, we don't pay enough attention to selecting them, and therefore, they can be either positive or negative. In fact, the very source of our low self-esteem is that we tend to repeat more negative affirmations than positive ones. Have you ever happened to say these sentences to yourself: "I can't do that"; "It won't work anyway"; "I have no power over it"; "They're better than me anyway"?

We need to know that, like every word, every thought has a certain level and degree of energy. Since an uttered word represents higher and more powerful energy than thought, every statement has a very significant energy content. Negative statements, by their very nature, carry negative energy, so their regular repetition results in the feeding of negative energies. Positive statements, on the other hand, are saturated with positive energy content, so if they are repeated systematically, we can reach positive energy multiplication. Positive affirmations are statements that describe the purpose we want to accomplish. These sentences, if repeated often, stimulate our minds. That's why it's essential to program your brain with positive affirmations. Our subconscious mind follows exactly what we say to it because it takes our words as commands. Give your brain positive instructions so that you will have a more successful life.

With the proper saturation of thought energy, the thought can materialize (come to fruition), whether positive or negative. A very good example is how Bonnie used to reject the offer of delicious food by saying, "I can't take it because of my eating problems!" As long she had such - surely negative - statements (about her overweight state), she indeed remained overweight. To make matters worse, by saying that one specific food makes us gain weight, we don't do anything other than putting its name into the "fattening" category. As a result of this negative programming, we will indeed gain weight.

Most people repeat the negative statements they create to bring about unwanted situations in their lives. The negative thoughts that we often say aloud are particularly dangerous because we gather negative energy when we think about events or things with a negative attitude. For example, when we are scared of something, we have no doubts about their realization, and therefore, we find it very plausible. As we perceive them realistically, we do not obstruct the realization of these thoughts. As a result, we are programming them into our subconscious.

—

How does it work?

This program is getting stored in the brain and, after frequent repetition by ourselves or others, is transformed into a reflex. We are particularly susceptible to this type of programming starting from our childhood when our unconscious mind is virtually a "clean sheet" and can accept or refuse anything. These programs become more and more intense as we practice our commentary during the years.

However, these words work not only in the wrong direction but also on the other side. Recognizing this, and especially applying it to our lives, can bring a qualitative change if we consciously use our positive thoughts. This form of behavior can change what we radiate, can improve our human relationships, and even our entire personality can become more positive. They can act as useful tools also in restoring self-confidence and self-esteem, so our quality of life can be significantly improved. Implementing the power of thought energy can help you achieve your goals. What happens when you have success at the psychological level? You can get closer to loving yourself and others, and thereby you can experience happiness, which is our purpose in life.

The good news is that one can achieve reprogramming bad runs and habits by applying cure-like positive reinforcements. Here is the recipe:

- Decide if you want to change.
- Recognize and record negative statements and indicators that adversely affect your life.
- Replace negative statements and adjectives with positive ones. For example, if you are having some issues with your weight, you probably tell yourself that "I can't resist food because I feel

---

69

terrible hunger." Replace this negative statement with the following, "Even when I am hungry, I am happy because I know I can do without food."

The daily use of affirmations seems endlessly simple, but we will often find that, despite our awareness, it does not work how we first imagined. Be persistent, and above all, be patient! Our bad habits and reflexes did not develop in a week, so it will take much more time to "reprogram" them. Until our positive reinforcements become reflexive, we must consciously observe they are correct to use. Practical implementation can be done in several ways. For one person, one method leads to a goal, while another person considers a different approach to be fool-proof. But, in our experience, it is most effective if the user recognizes its importance, fully accepts the method, and feels no internal resistance or doubts while using it. Reinforcements work most effectively when used in the present tense with singular first person, e.g., "I can do it!" Why don't I recommend using future tense? Because we take the risk that our brain won't move immediately in the desired direction, as procrastination is part of human nature!

You can improve the effectiveness of your reinforcements by pronouncing them aloud with a positive, confident, and emphatic charge. In some cases, you can practice it with the silent method as well, if the background voice is not excessive, but beware of repeating them only in your head. The point is that statements should always be persuasive and transmit determination. You can record the reinforcements that you think are good, with pre-planned exercises at the same time and place every day. You can use any appropriate situation during the day to accomplish this task. For example, you can practice during a trip or a boring meeting. The bottom line is, practice every day! It would be super-efficient if you could say your positive affirmations several times a day. However, they will work in your favor only if you don't consider it obligatory, but voluntary to improve your life. Know that, like anyone else, you can direct your actions positively through your positive thoughts, and in that way, change your quality of life in a positive direction and make yourself happier.

The most effective method to Use Affirmations

A few people say assertions for all to hear before a mirror. Others essentially record them in a diary. You can likewise rehash them in your mind like a mantra during contemplation.

The significant thing is to discover assertions that impact you. I'll concede that there are a lot of confirmations out there that are simply to charm for me and don't impact me. Now and then, individuals toss in words like "show" and "plenitude," however, these words just don't impact me (yet perhaps they accomplish for you!).

Weight reduction insistences are an extraordinary approach to motivate your excursion toward your weight reduction. You can utilize these positive attestations for getting thinner to help program your psyche with positive propensities.

We as a whole know weight reduction isn't about that simple. We are utilizing these weight reduction assertions can even assistance the individuals who face difficult inward opposition when attempting to thin down. This article will furnish you with a rundown of positive certifications for getting in shape and construct certainty.

Benefits of Positive Affirmation

Positive affirmation isn't just the act of trying to "fake it 'til you make it." Rather, positive affirmation is the act of focusing on positive values, making you more resilient to stress and other gunk you don't need in your life. If that alone doesn't convince you, here are some more benefits positive affirmation could give you:

- Positive affirmation lets you see the water in the half-filled glass – going back to the analogy of the pessimist and the optimist, and the optimist will be able to water a wilting plant, quench someone's thirst, clean something, etc. with the water that he sees. The pessimist, on the other hand, sees nothing but the lack of water to fill the cup and does nothing until the remaining amount of water completely evaporates. Using the power of affirmation, you open up worlds of possibilities you never thought existed, which will definitely give you more opportunities to do things that make you happy.

- Positive affirmation gives you control over your life – by practicing positive affirmation, you will have much better control over different aspects of your life simply because you're more aware of events that hurt you and events that help you and are consciously making an effort to choose the latter.

- Positive affirmation doesn't have to be a mundane ritual – positive affirmation isn't just for helping you make great company presentations or helping you overcome stress; positive affirmation is also for helping you achieve new goals and dreams! You can positively affirm yourself with a power chant or even a power stance to enforce your ideas. In a sense, positive affirmation is already a positive event in your daily routine!

Chapter 14. Positive Affirmations For Weight Loss

When you start losing weight, whether, for health or aesthetic reasons, it is not always easy to stay in the long term, thanks to positive affirmations, we will be able to gain motivation and self-esteem. What are positive affirmations? To make positive affirmations is to speak to yourself, out loud

The positive affirmations for losing weight are, therefore, daily support and easy to set up, allowing to continue the work done in the session. They allow you to work on both self-esteem and self-confidence, which are essential on the path to weight loss.

The positive affirmations to lose weight that we use are therefore linked to self-love. Taking extra adoration of your body and your food is an act of self-love. Looking at yourself in the mirror and telling yourself how wonderful you are is a great positive message that you give yourself. It can all start with just smiling at yourself. So whatever way you plan to lose weight or even free yourself from compulsions, give yourself this kindness. Because you just deserve it!

- Getting thinner easily falls into place for me.
- I am joyfully accomplishing my weight reduction objectives.
- I am getting thinner consistently.
- I love to practice routinely.
- I am eating nourishments that adds to my wellbeing and prosperity.
- I eat just when I am ravenous.

- I presently unmistakably observe myself at my optimal weight.

- I love the flavor of sound food.

- I am in charge of the amount I eat.

- I am getting a charge out of working out; it causes me to feel great.

- I am turning out to be fitter and more grounded ordinarily through exercise.

- I am effectively reaching and keep up my optimal weight

- I love and care for my body.

- I have the right to have a thin, solid, appealing body.

- I am growing increasingly good dieting propensities constantly.

- I am getting slimmer consistently.

- I look and feel extraordinary.

- I take the necessary steps to be sound.

- I am joyfully re-imagined achievement.

- I decide to work out.

- I need to eat nourishments that cause me to look and feel great.

- I am answerable for my wellbeing.

- I love my body.

- I am quiet with making my better body.

- I am joyfully practicing each morning when I wake up with the goal that I can arrive at the weight reduction that I have been needing.
- I am subscribing to my get-healthy plan by changing my dietary patterns from undesirable to solid.
- I am content with each part I do in my incredible exertion to shed pounds.
- Consistently I am getting slimmer and more advantageous.
- I am building up an appealing body.
- I am building up a way of life of energetic wellbeing.
- I am making a body that I like and appreciate.
- My way of life eating changes is changing my body.
- I am feeling incredible since I have lost more than 10 pounds in about a month and can hardly wait to meet my woman companion.
- I have a level stomach.
- I commend my own capacity to settle on decisions around food.
- I am joyfully gauging 20 pounds less.
- I am cherishing strolling 3 to 4 times each week and do conditioning practices, in any event, three times each week
- I drink eight glasses of water a day.
- I eat products of the soil every day and generally eat chicken and fish.

- I am learning and utilizing the psychological, passionate, and otherworldly aptitudes for progress. I will change it!
- I will make new musings about my self and my body.
- I adore and value my body.
- It's energizing to find my exceptional food and exercise framework for weight reduction.
- I am a weight reduction example of overcoming adversity.
- I am enchanted to be the perfect load for me.
- It's simple for me to follow a sound food plan.
- I decided to grasp the musings of trust in my capacity to roll out positive improvements throughout my life.
- It feels great to move my body. Exercise is entertaining!
- I utilize profound breathing to assist me with unwinding and handle the pressure.
- I am a wonderful individual.
- I have the right to be at my optimal weight.
- I am an adorable individual. I merit love. It is alright for me to shed pounds.
- I am a solid nearness on the planet at my lower weight.
- I discharge the need to blame my body.
- I acknowledge and make the most of my sexuality. It's OK to feel sexy.
- My digestion is brilliant.
- I keep up my body with ideal wellbeing.

- I love my body likes to be healthy My heart is from the center of love
- I love every cell in my body; I move comfortably and easily. My feet will dance through life. I know how to care for myself. I am in good shape and health than I have ever been
- I love my beautiful body " We agree that positive affirmations are not enough.
- I deserve to have the body I want
- I take care of myself, and it makes me feel good
- I feel better and better
- I am proud not to give in to gluttony, bad for my health
- Each day brings me a little closer to my goal
- I have a healthy life, and I eliminate my bad habits
- I lose weight because I love myself (not because I don't like my body)
- I am deserving of happiness and to have confidence in myself
- I can do it
- My body needs better from me.
- I have the right to be solid and fit as a fiddle.
- Rationalizing consumes zero calories for each hour.
- Getting fit as a fiddle is something I can achieve.
- Getting fit as a fiddle is fundamental for a long healthy life

Chapter 15. Positive Affirmations for Healing and Health

- I choose to heal.
- I believe in my ability to manifest happiness and healing.
- My health is improving.
- My body is healing itself.
- The body I have keeps getting stronger each day.
- I am healed.
- I am in great shape.
- I am grateful for my body and what it can do.
- I am listening to my body and meet its needs.
- I am improving the state of my body every day.
- I am healed, healthy, happy, and free of pain
- I enjoy playing in my own vessel, and I am grateful that I no longer have back pain.
- I am healthy, happy, and thriving.
- I enjoy feeling healthy, and I am grateful that my back is healed and free from pain.
- I appreciate my healthy mind, body, and spirit.
- My back is strong, healthy, flexible, and free of pain.
- I am psyched. I am healthy, happy, and I am not experiencing back pain.
- I am not suffering from back pain, and I have gratefulness.
- I am healthy, happy, and in harmony.

- My body is in good health and free from pain.
- My spirit, mind, and body are in harmony, healthy, and happy. I am pain-free
- I am pain-free, happy, and healthy.
- My back is healthy and pain-free.
- I will do important steps in healing my back. These steps help me to be free from pain
- I am moving with freedom and joy in my body.
- I am enjoying my healthy body and am free of any and all residual pain.
- I have the tools needed to heal my body. For this, I am grateful.
- The body I have is free of pain; I am moving through life with grace and joy
- I am glad to be completely pain-free.
- My back is flexible and strong. I walk with grace and ease.
- I am choosing a life that does not include having pain, only happiness, and good health
- I enjoy my pain-free back and my pain-free body.
- I have gratefulness for my healthy pain-free back and body.
- My body is healthy and thriving.
- I have the right to have good health, and I am happy with my body, not feeling pain.
- I am in control of my life.
- I willingly take my power back.
- I permit myself to heal.

- I release everything which I don`t need.
- I choose to focus on my recovery and healing.
- I am attracting good health.
- I respect my body.
- I am confident and comfortable with my body.
- I love myself and my body.
- I am grateful for the body I have.
- My body is resilient and strong.
- My body has it's own unique beauty.
- I will only consume nourishing foods into my body.
- I am grateful for the strength and power my body possesses.
- My body is my vessel.
- I look and feel youthful.
- I am gracefully aging.
- For the entirety of my life, I am choosing good health.
- I am embracing the wisdom of the body I am blessed with
- I take care of the vessel or body I have.
- I have a feeling of gratefulness for great health at every stage of my life.
- I choose healthy foods for good health
- I choose healing foods for the nourishment of my body
- I am letting go of the emotion that is making habits that are unhealthy.
- I love eating healthy foods.

- I choose to eat healthy foods.
- My body is indulging on all the nutrients and vitamins it needs
- I will only eat foods that are beneficial to me.
- My body is fit and strong.
- I am choosing wellbeing because I need it
- I nourish my mind, body, and soul every day.
- My body and mind are vibrant and healthy.
- I am radiating joy, confidence, and health.
- My immune system is healthy and strong.
- The body I have is in optimum shape.
- My mind is calm and at peace.
- The source will flow through my body
- I have gratefulness to be here on earth
- I am happy and excited at the moment
- I am full of energy.
- I find energy in purposeful work.
- I align my goals with the radiating energy the Cosmos is giving me
- Life is beautiful and amazing.
- I am healed.
- My body is becoming stronger, and it is healing quickly.
- The immune system I have is working to heal my body.
- I have perfect health.
- I have a healing energy surrounding me.

- My health is becoming better as each day goes by.
- I am whole and healthy.
- I am feeling the happiness of being alive.
- Good health and joy fill my everyday life.
- Good energy is flowing through my body freely
- I am radiating vitality and positive energy.
- My life is full of health and happiness.
- I feel excited to start my day with a smile.

Chapter 16. Positive Affirmations for Positivity and Self-Esteem

A great way to raise your self-esteem is through the use of affirmations. The regular practice of affirmations can help us to change our beliefs about life and ourselves and thereby reprogram our minds. If you have low self-esteem, it's mostly a product of conscious or unconscious programming during your childhood by your family, friends, teachers, society, the media, and even by yourself.

By repeating positive statements many times, a day, you convince your subconscious mind to believe them. Once your subconscious mind is convinced, you start acting accordingly. You start believing you are a person with high self-esteem, and then you become it. Yes, it really is that simple. You have to practice a lot, though. Affirmations help you develop the mentality, thoughts, and beliefs you need to take your self-esteem to the next level. I highly recommend writing down your affirmations and reading them out loud various times daily.

It's important to state them positively and in the present so that your subconscious mind can't differentiate between if it's already true or "only" imagined. Affirmations do have to be personal, positively stated, specific, emotionally charged, and in the present tense. Here are some examples:

The more you are practicing, the better you are getting at it. The first time you say, "I'm a person with healthy self-esteem and happy about it," your inner voice will still say, "No, you are not. You are small, and you have no right to happiness." However, after repeating it 200 times

84

every day for a week, you should have silenced your inner critic. Make your affirmations your permanent company. Repeat them as often as you like, and have a look at what happens in your life.

Nevertheless, some studies claim that affirmations actually have negative effects on people with very low self-esteem. If your inner critic just doesn't get convinced, if you notice no benefit at all, or if things get worse instead of better - which happens in very few cases - try other techniques like subliminal tapes (they go directly to your subconscious without any chance of self-judgment) or ask yourself other questions such as "Why am I so happy? Why is everything working out?" Did you just notice? When you ask a question, the inner critic stays quiet. Instead of self-talking you down, your mind is now searching for answers to the question you asked

You have come a long way, and I want you to confirm these affirmations with yourself frequently. Remember to choose a comfortable space to sit in. Perhaps a space that allows you to speak out loud now. Keep your breathing exercises in mind, always maintaining an even rhythm in your breathing. This is a fun exercise, an exercise that will reassure you of your worth. Now, allow me to guide you.

I want you to participate in this part by repeating my words. Please do repeat these words out loud because it's essential to hear your own voice. I will pause briefly after each affirmation, and you will have the time to repeat the sentence. Shall we begin?

- I deserve to be happy and successful.
- I am competent, smart, and able.
- Every day and in every way I'm feeling better and better

- I love the person I am becoming.

- I follow up with everything I say and do.

- I acknowledge my own value, and my confidence continues to grow each day.

- I strongly believe in my own abilities and skills to attract a positive outcome.

- I am fully capable of reaching any target I set for myself with my newfound confidence.

- I will aim to make memories I treasure because I refuse to live a robotic life.

- I will walk into the spotlight with my head held high because I no longer fear the crowd.

- I'm not afraid of meeting new people because I'm interesting and have so much to offer.

- I don't need to compare myself to another person because I'm unique.

- I have the confidence to speak to anyone because my voice is a powerful tool.

- I'm confident in my knowledge and refuse to doubt my own words.

- I will take some brief time off now and then because life can become hectic for anyone.

- I will finish my tasks one by one and not become overwhelmed.

- I will own my mistakes instead of punishing myself.

- I'm a powerful force, and nothing in the world can shove me off track.
- I will not allow myself to take on more than I can handle.
- I acknowledge the fact that I cannot control everything.
- I acknowledge that I'm not perfect because no person is.
- I won't allow my fears to control my thinking and prevent me from living life to the fullest.
- I have complete control over negative emotions that plague me at night.
- I will create what is best for me because I control my imagination.
- I am strong enough to defeat any addiction or pain.
- I'm a strong, confident, kind, and loving person who is capable of anything I set my mind to.

Chapter 17. Rules of Repetition

The brain adores repetition since its recognizable - and natural is ameliorating. One reason repetition works are for a similar explanation - the dull hypnotic recommendation gets comfortable to the customer, and they arrive at a more in-depth condition of hypnosis as the conscious mind unwinds into a feeling of 'ah we've heard this previously.'

This makes the hypnosis meeting increasingly charming and compelling for the customer and causes them to accomplish a more prominent degree of achievement quicker. With proceeded with repetition of original proposals previously, during, and after the hypnosis meeting, the recommendation turns out to be recognizable to the point that it becomes what we call a propensity for the mind - or what I like to request an executable program of the brain.

Repetition is perhaps the most straightforward approach to persuade individuals regarding something. At the point when we hear things on different occasions, we will, in general, trust it more. It turns out to be increasingly natural, and progressively recognizable things appear to be all the more evident. Yet, we must have an original contention and realities to back our situation up, isn't that right? Also, we should have the other individual's consideration!

Repetition rule

Rule: If something happens frequently enough, I will, in the long run, be convinced.

How it functions

Play it once more, Sam. Music rehashed gets under our skin. Commercials rehashed replay themselves when we see the item. Repetition of things distinctly affects us.

Example

Our brains are great example matches and prize us for utilizing this accommodating ability. Repetition makes an example, which, therefore, and catches our eye typically from the outset and afterward makes the solace of commonality.

Recognition

Repetition makes a recognition, yet does commonality breed disdain? Even though it can occur, actually commonality prompts preferring in undeniably more cases than it does to hatred. At the point when we are in a grocery store, we are unmistakably bound to purchase natural brands, regardless of whether we have never attempted the item. Sponsors know this well indeed.

Not shortage

An impact that can happen is that repetition nullifies any shortage impact, making something at first less alluring. At the point when I work with a well-an individual, my underlying condition overawed may before long be supplanted by the aversion of their irritating propensities. With time, in any case (if they are not very repulsive), I will presumably become acclimated to them and even get the opportunity to acknowledge and like the better pieces of their temperament.

Understanding

Repetition can likewise prompt comprehension, as it gives time for the penny to drop. What form might the outset be abnormal after rehashed presentation turns out to be clear and reasonable?

This is significant for organizations carrying inventive new items to the market where clients may look at first new to the item or its use.

Memory

Recall learning your augmentation tables at junior school? We need to rehash things more than once for them to at last sink into our recollections. Our transient memories are famously present moment and can overlook something (like an individual's name) in under a second. Repetition is often one of the things into longer-term memory and is also an essential technique for learning.

Persuading

A few people simply need to do things a few times before they decide. Consider the last time you purchased a couple of shoes. Did you pick them at that point put them da few times before giving them a shot? Did you return to attempt them once more? Assuming this is the case, you are following after some admirable people. Numerous individuals need to rehash things a few times before they get persuaded. Multiple times is an average number.

Bothering

We can likewise get convinced in a negative redundant manner. All youngsters realize that if they rehash a solicitation frequently enough, their folks will collapse. Some recollect this when they grow up and get hitched - the annoying mate is an incredible symbol.

Daze

Repetition is additionally a reason for daze states and is like this a premise of hypnosis and hypnotic procedures.

At the point when you are figuring out how to do self-hypnosis, you'll have to utilize hypnosis contents to achieve the objectives you have set out for yourself. Through hypnosis, you will find the capacity to improve numerous parts of your life. Materials will permit you to arrive at your subconscious mind with positive affirmations and repetition.

When utilizing content for hypnosis, it's critical to use them absolutely. Negative articulations will make your mind see the exercises you are attempting to stop before it sees your messages to change. You would fortify the very propensities you are endeavoring to prevent. Instead of utilizing contrary explanations, use invigorating, positive articulations that will point your subconscious the correct way.

Your contents ought to likewise be in the dynamic or current state, without reference to the past. You can't change the past; you are attempting to change what will occur later on. Abstain from utilizing action words that identify with the past tense. Keeping your announcements clear, positive, and straightforward will provide your precise subconscious orders, which it would then be able to follow.

Self-hypnosis causes you to make recommendations that will influence your subconscious mind for it to work, you should rehash your proposals with the goal that you'll be engraving these on your subconscious mind. It might likewise be useful to go astray from your set expressions once in for a little while, utilizing somewhat various words to affirm similar expectations.

A dynamic and definite methodology will help put you out and about toward your objectives. In case you're attempting to shed pounds, for instance, you may express that you are shedding pounds every day to arrive at your objective weight objective. Give yourself a timetable to work with, and show your goal plainly. If you simply represent that you will get in shape, it doesn't set a definite intention before you. You can customize your content by continually utilizing "I" instead of "you." This will assist with making them increasingly viable. Repeating your announcements unobtrusively using the pronoun "I" will better affect your subconscious.

Actual contents are useful to increase the comprehension of how you can give yourself proposals. Your proposals ought to be valuable for you and novel to your motivations. The contents you use will assist you with utilizing and comprehend the different ways you can speak with your subconscious mind.

Utilizing sentences of fluctuating lengths can help make your objectives understood to your subconscious mind. Longer sentences are more earnestly for your mind to see, so don't utilize excessively protracted phrases. Short and medium proclamations will shield your content from appearing to be repetitive.

Self-hypnosis can push you to reconstruct your mind successfully by directly talking with your subconscious. Your subconscious mind puts together its musings with respect to your feelings. You can change your temperament and adjust your conduct or propensities if you use contents in a positive and re-confirming way. Utilizing legitimate proclamations for your hypnosis contents is fundamental to arriving at your objective.

Chapter 18. The Power of Repeated Words and Thoughts

Auto-conditioning is like broadcasting to yourself. It consists of three basic steps. First, in able for one to converse with their subconscious successfully, one must do some diversion to the conscious mind so that it presents as little resistance if possible This is commonly done by producing some peaceful attitude, the method of how you relax in a comfortable chair when you are watching the television Second, you must convince the subconscious that what it thinks it likes, it should really dislike. This you do by actually talking to yourself—out loud or silently, through visualization. Finally, you must encourage the subconscious to what your conscious intelligence knows to be beneficial. The readiness of the subconscious to obey implicitly is the secret of the success of this method. Another built-in success factor is the progressive ease with which auto-conditioning is accomplished. Each time you relax and talk to yourself, it happens more quickly and more effectively. You can actually deepen your relaxation with practice to the point where it can be called a pleasant trance-like state. In this state, your subconscious is practically naked to the spoken word, ready to do your intelligent bidding.

Part of that bidding can be to deepen the state, even more, the next time. The following session, without even trying, you will sink more quickly into an even deeper state of receptivity. As sure as the conditioned reflex, you will make even greater strides in molding your eating habits to be automatically perfect for you without strain, win power or effort. Self-hypnosis, or auto-conditioning, becomes easier and easier. First, you may induce relaxation by counting from one to ten. Later, you can count by two's—two, four, six, eight, ten—and reach the relaxed state in double-quick time. Finally, you will be able to command yourself to assume the relaxed state merely by thinking of the number ten.

Talk yourself thin, and you stay thin. You are not on another fad to trim the fat. Auto-conditioning is the ultimate method to grow and stay slender because it changes the very mechanism that has motivated you to eat fat-producing foods. It spells the end in your life of painful poundage and the beginning of new-found youth, health, and vigor. However, it is not like a pill that can be downed with a gulp of water. To begin this method and follow it through takes conviction.

How it works the idea of talking to the subconscious can present a block to many people. Are you talking to some automaton, some robot, some entity other than yourself? The answer is no. Your subconscious is most definitely you. When you talk to your subconscious, you are talking to yourself. (Italicized you and yourself will be used in the topics ahead in place of the word "subconscious." You and yourself will be the person you, your family, and friends know you to be. You and yourself will be the slave and master that remembers all, obeys implicitly and controls you.) You can talk to yourself right now. Say, "I hate cake!" Say it either out loud or silently. Say it again. Now again. You have said it three times. Of course, you still like cake. But one thing is sure: you don't have it more than you did a minute ago, and very likely the next time you face up to cake, you will remember this moment. If you were placed in a state of hypnosis and told three times that cake tastes as bad to you like some food for which you cherish a particular dislike, you would not be likely to eat cake again. The method of talking to yourself taught you in this guide is a form of self-hypnosis, better known as auto-conditioning. The success rate will be depending on a great deal on how closely you follow the relaxation techniques described in the topics ahead. Exposing your subconscious to your suggestion is the key. Using imagery while the subconscious is exposed is the basic technique. What is the imagery? You use it every day without being consciously aware of it. Try it now.

Here is how you can practice. Get some white cards or small white sheets of scratch paper. Draw a circle in pencil. Try holding this for about one foot in front of your eyes. Stare at it. Now close your eyes. Try to picture it. Can you imagine how it looks? Now draw a square. Close your eyes and picture it. Then put the square in the circle. Try to visualize that. Now without actually drawing the square's diagonals, close your eyes and visualize the square inside the circle with diagonal corners connected by crossing lines. You will be using this power of imagining to picture yourself the attractive, slender person you are going to be. It will help you get there faster. Begin this imagining now by looking at your face in the mirror. Then close your eyes and try to see your face. Was your hair combed? Did a double chin show? Now picture your hair groomed just the way you want it. Picture the chin firm and youthful. Do this habitually, and you will see for yourself that you are paying more attention to the hair. What about the chin? There will be some surprises there, too!

Properly receptive, your subconscious will respond automatically. You will eat with gusto just what you have instructed yourself to enjoy. You will turn away effortlessly from what you are not supposed to enjoy. You will be on a permanent diet without knowing it. You will be able to pass up a pie a la mode and never feel deprived. You will eat fruit and gelatin desserts and savor them as much as baked Alaska. As the days go by, the scale will register, increasing weight losses. You will be surprised every time you step on the scale. You have not dieted through painful self-discipline. Yet you will lose as much weight as if you had followed those typewritten diet sheets religiously. Without the pain of deprivation, the days will add up to weeks faster, and the weeks will fly by faster. Two pounds or more a week will soon register 10, 20, 30 pounds off on the scale! There is no limit to the weight you can safely lose by talking yourself thin, as compared to other more difficult methods. Once you attain your normal weight, there's no diet to stop, no process to reverse. You stay thin — naturally. It's as simple as that!

Chapter 19. Hypnosis and Mind

Hypnosis is a state of receptivity. When a person is in a state of hypnosis, they are more open to suggestions and messages were given by the hypnotist. The suggestions, within reason, are not analyzed by the conscious mind, but the subconscious mind accepts them. Once messages go into the subconscious mind, they become automatic and natural responses.

This altered state happens naturally throughout the day. Anytime you zone out, daydream, or even go into a deep state of focused concentration, you go into a state similar to hypnosis! You also pass into a hypnotic state as you are falling asleep at night, and when awakening in the morning. The average person is not aware they are more receptive as they are waking up or falling asleep. Hence, they usually overlook the benefits of using these naturally occurring receptive states.

It is a fact that once an idea gets implanted into the subconscious mind, it stays there until a new one replaces it. The longer an idea remains in your subconscious mind, the harder it becomes to replace it with a new one.

The process of hypnosis strives to UNLOCK your subconscious mind This is how hypnosis works. It attempts to replace your old thought patterns with new ones to change the basic way your subconscious and the conscious mind works.

Hypnosis works by bringing the action of this subconscious to the forefront and gives the control of our conscious mind the backseat. It clears all the clutter that might cloud your conscious mind and makes way for the subconscious to accept new thoughts and ideas.

The conscious and subconscious mind

For you to be able to understand how to hypnotize someone, it's first important to know that the concept of hypnosis is entirely based on the intricate relationship between the conscious and subconscious mind.

In our everyday lives, we seem to be in total control of our conscious minds. In other words, it appears to us that we use our conscious minds to think and make decisions. Meanwhile, we tend to think of our subconscious mind as a dormant part of our brain, not having much to do with our everyday functioning.

However, the opposite is true. It is the subconscious mind that is controlling the actions of our conscious mind. In fact, our subconscious mind is the most automatic part of our brain, the one who controls most of our life processes, including emotions, reflexes, automatic behavior, belief systems, and even breathing. Above all, our subconscious mind is responsible for how we perceive the world around us, how our body processes the physical information it receives, and how our key thought processes are formed.

You must understand the difference between conscious communication and subconscious communication. The conscious part of the mind is a very analytical, logical, critical part of the mind where information is analyzed. However, to change a person's habits, patterns, beliefs, feelings, sensations, emotions, etc., we want to get into the subconscious part of the mind. We do this by bypassing the conscious, analytical, critical mind. The way that you'll be learning how to do this is with hypnotic communication will allow you to connect with anyone hypnotically, so what you say will bypass the critical mind and get directly into the powerful and natural subconscious mind.

Conscious Versus Subconscious Communication

The conscious mind is the very logical and analytical part of the mind. The last thing you want is for your target to be analyzing every word that comes out of your mouth. The more people overanalyze what you are saying, the more they have a chance to build doubt, fear, resistance, and objections against you. The subconscious is the piece of the mind that stores all of your experiences and also composes your thoughts, feelings, emotions, behaviors, feelings, and habits. We want to communicate with that part of the mind so we can bypass any analytical thinking, knock down any resistance, and build trust with our target. When you communicate directly to the subconscious mind, the target is more likely to accept what you say as the truth because you are evoking emotions, feelings, and sensations that can influence their behaviors, habits, and decisions. That can be used in any sales situation or relationship.

Upon first learning how to connect with someone hypnotically, sometimes people think they will use their voice or their words to zap a person into a trance. However, there is much more than just hypnotic language, although you will learn a lot of hypnotic language in this guide.

The Critical Factor

In your pursuit of learning how to hypnotize someone, you will need to master the art of bypassing the critical factor in your subject's mind.

The critical factor is a part of the conscious mind which stands like a filter between it and the subconscious. It has the ability to accept or reject any new stimulus, such as ideas or thoughts that might want to enter

---

99

your conscious mind from the subconscious. The basic duty of the critical factor is to protect our minds from any threats and dangers. By design, our nervous system views change and new ideas as a threat. Hence, any new stimulus is not likely to be seen as a part of our existing mental set-up. As a result, the critical factor rejects such inputs from the subconscious, thus preventing change.

The process of hypnosis helps to quiet down the critical factor for a short while, clearing the way for passage of new ideas from the subconscious to the conscious mind.

Bypassing the Critical Factor

How to communicate to the subconscious mind is through a process called "bypassing the critical factor of the conscious mind." The critical factor is like a filter that keeps information from getting to the subconscious mind unless it belongs there. When this filter is bypassed (or lowered), it can form new habits or programs, evoke emotional states, or influence a belief or the way we perceive something.

These four ways to bypass the critical factor are:

1. Heightened Emotional States

Anytime you experience a heightened emotional state, your guard is lowered, and information naturally enters the subconscious mind. This is often how fears and anxieties form. Fear is a heightened emotional state where a person can experience a fight or flight response. Negative emotions will usually result in a negative mismatched program that forms In the same way that negative emotions bypass the critical factor of the conscious mind to form new programs, positive emotions will have a similar effect. When people experience positive emotions, though, they will often feel good about the decisions they are making, and the people around them. Therefore, it is crucial that in your communication strategies, to build the "know, like, and trust factor," you evoke positive emotions in your target. Imagine if you are selling your services or product to them, and they are feeling happy and excited about it, they will feel much better about listening to you, and the resistance goes down. When you evoke positive emotions, you can also get people to make decisions faster and easier, feel better about the decision they are making, and have their choice benefit both you and them.

2. Repetition Is the Mother of All Learning

You may have heard this before: "repetition is the mother of all learning." This statement is true. Every time something is repeated, it knocks on the critical factor until it lowers that guard and gets into your subconscious mind. That is why advertisers say it takes 7 to 11 repetitions of a message for a target or prospect to take action or decide about the product. Think about things you just do naturally, habits, or behaviors you have that you don't even have to think about anymore. Brushing your teeth, tying your shoes, opening a door, driving a car. You don't have to sit there every time you open a door and analyze how to do it, do you? Of course, not! You have repeated that action or behavior so often that it becomes a natural part of your powerful subconscious mind. That is why you should use the repetition of a message when communicating with your target. Often, people will misinterpret this principle and think they must repeat the same sentence or phrase repeatedly. Still, you don't have to use the same sentence or phrase over again, and you can use the repetition of a concept or idea conveyed in different ways.

Think of jingles or product slogans you hear on the radio or television. As soon as a commercial play, they have a jingle associated with a particular product, so when you hear the jingle, you think of the product. That is due to having listened to that jingle several times. That is also why in commercials and advertisements, you will often hear phone numbers, websites, or services repeated at least three times. It creates a link in your memory with the information they want you to record and remember.

3. Authority and Credibility

There are just some people that we build such a high level of respect or trust in that everything they say is held in high regard. That is often true with religious figures. When people enter a church, synagogue, temple, or any other religious institution, our critical factor becomes bypassed. The same thing is valid with parents, coaches, doctors, and some political figures. Without getting controversial here, if you want to see a great example of mass hypnosis, the next time you walk into a church, and everyone stands and sings at the same time, ask yourself, "Am I hypnotized?" Authority figures set our expectations, condition our beliefs, and will often influence our behaviors.

How do you use this method in your communication with your target? It's quite simple! Use certificates, social proof, testimonials, and newspaper clippings to position yourself as the obvious expert in your industry. Imagine walking into a doctor's office, and seeing a wall lined with degrees and certificates, you immediately establish more trust in that doctor because their degrees and certificates are usually an indication of their credentials. That is also why referrals work. Think about it. Someone who you trust is giving you a referral, and that creates an expectation that the professional you will hire will do a good job. It's the same if your friends set you up with someone to go on a date. They may say, "Oh, you'll love this person!" That sets up an expectation based on the credibility of your friends.

4. Conventional Hypnosis Versus Hypnotic Communication

With conventional hypnotism, you're putting somebody into a trancelike state. They are willing participants, and we use that trancelike state to change a behavior, feeling emotion, or habit. We evoke this trancelike state by applying a hypnotic induction. The hypnotic induction bypasses the conscious mind and allows the hypnotic suggestions to be accepted as if they were real.

That brings up the ethical and moral obligations and issues again. However, please know that it is very complicated and near impossible to get a person to do something that they would not be willing to do. However, think of a family member for whom you would do anything or another person with whom you have a meaningful connection. What lengths would you go to for that person? These connections and techniques can have a very similar effect.

Chapter 20. Hypnosis and Weight Loss

Hypnosis plays an important role in medicinal solutions. In modern-day society, it is recommended for treating many different conditions, including obesity or weight loss, in individuals who are overweight. It also serves patients who have undergone surgery extremely well, particularly if they are restricted from exercising after surgery. Given that it is the perfect option for losing weight, it is additionally helpful to anyone who is disabled or recovering from an injury.

Once you understand the practice and how it is conducted, you will find that everything makes sense. Hypnosis works for weight loss because of the relationship between our minds and bodies. Without proper communication being relayed from our minds to our bodies, we would not be able to function properly. Since hypnosis allows the brain to adopt new ideas and habits, it can help push anyone in the right direction and could potentially improve our quality of living.

Hypnosis is a practice used for losing weight, but since healing forms an essential part of retraining both the body and mind to perform in perfect harmony, it needs to be treated as a tool to calm the mind. Once you've mastered the art of self-control, you can move on and easily convince yourself that you are capable of losing weight, reaching your goal weight, and achieving many other fitness goals that you once thought wasn't possible.

Losing weight with hypnosis works just like any other change with hypnosis will. However, it is important to understand the step by step process so that you know exactly what to expect during your weight loss journey with the support of hypnosis. In general, there are about seven steps that are involved with weight loss using hypnosis. The first step is when you decide to change; the second step involves your sessions; the third and fourth are your changed mindset and behaviors, the fifth step involves your regressions, the sixth is your management routines, and the seventh is your lasting change. To give you a clearer idea of what each of these parts of your journey looks like, let's explore them in greater detail below.

In your first step toward achieving weight loss with hypnosis, you have decided that you desire change and that you are willing to try hypnosis as a way to change your approach to weight loss. At this point, you have an awareness of the fact that you want to lose weight, and you have been shown the possibility of losing weight through hypnosis. You may find yourself feeling curious, open to trying something new, and a little bit skeptical as to whether or not this is going to work for you. You may also be feeling frustrated, overwhelmed, or even defeated by the lack of success you have seen using other weight loss methods, which may be what lead you to seek out hypnosis in the first place. At this stage, the best thing you can do is practice keeping an open and curious mind, as this is how you can set yourself up for success when it comes to your actual hypnosis sessions.

Your sessions account for stage two of the process. Technically, you are going to move from stage two through to stage five several times over before you officially move into stage six. Your sessions are the stage where you engage in hypnosis, nothing more, and nothing less. During your sessions, you need to maintain your open mind and stay focused on how hypnosis can help you. If you are struggling to stay open-minded or are still skeptical about how this might work, you can consider switching from absolute confidence that it will help to have a curiosity about how it might help instead.

Following your sessions, you are first going to experience a changed mindset. This is where you start to feel far more confident in your ability to lose weight and in your ability to keep the weight off. At first, your mindset may still be shadowed by doubt, but as you continue to use hypnosis and see your results, you will realize that you can create success with hypnosis. As these pieces of evidence start to show up in your own life, you will find your hypnosis sessions becoming even more powerful and even more successful.

In addition to a changed mindset, you are going to start to see changed behaviors. They may be smaller at first, but you will find that they increase over time until they reach the point where your behaviors reflect exactly the lifestyle you have been aiming to have. The best part about these changed behaviors is that they will not feel forced, nor will they feel like you have had to encourage yourself to get here: your changed mindset will make these changed behaviors incredibly easy for you to choose. As you continue working on your hypnosis and experiencing your changed mind, you will find that your behavioral changes grow more significant and more effortless every single time.

Following your hypnosis and your experiences with changed mindset and behaviors, you are likely going to experience regression periods. Regression periods are characterized by periods where you begin to engage in your old mindset and behavior once again. This happens because you have experienced this old mindset and behavioral patterns so many times over that they continue to have deep roots in your subconscious mind. The more you uproot them and reinforce your new behaviors with consistent hypnosis sessions, the more success you will have in eliminating these old behaviors and replacing them entirely with new ones. Anytime you experience the beginning of a regression period, you should set aside some time to engage in a hypnosis session to help you shift your mindset back into the state that you want.

Your management routines account for the sixth step, and they come into place after you have effectively experienced a significant and lasting change from your hypnosis practices. At this point, there's no need to schedule as frequent of hypnosis sessions because you are experiencing such significant changes in your mindset. However, you may still want to do hypnosis sessions on a fairly consistent basis to ensure that your mindset remains changed and that you do not revert into old patterns. Sometimes, it can take up to 3-6 months or longer with these consistent management routine hypnosis sessions to maintain your changes and prevent you from experiencing a significant regression in your mindset and behavior.

The final step in your hypnosis journey is going to be the step where you come upon lasting changes. At this point, you are unlikely to need to schedule hypnosis sessions any longer. You should not need to rely on hypnosis at all to change your mindset because you have experienced such significant changes already, and you no longer find yourself regressing into old behaviors. With that being said, you may find that from time to time, you need to have a hypnosis session just to maintain your changes, particularly when an unexpected trigger may arise that may cause you to want to regress your behaviors. These unexpected changes can happen for years following your successful changes, so staying on top of them and relying on your healthy coping method of hypnosis is important as it will prevent you from experiencing a significant regression later in life.

Using hypnosis to encourage healthy eating and discourage unhealthy eating

As you go through using hypnosis to support you with weight loss, there are a few ways that you are going to do so. One of the ways is to focus on weight loss. Another way, however, is to focus on topics surrounding weight loss. For example, you can use hypnosis to help you encourage yourself to eat healthy while also helping discourage yourself from unhealthy eating. Effective hypnosis sessions can help you bust cravings for foods that are going to sabotage your success while also helping you feel more drawn to making choices that are going to help you effectively lose weight.

Many people will use hypnosis as a way to change their cravings, improve their metabolism, and even help themselves acquire a taste for eating healthier foods. You may also use this to help encourage you to develop the motivation and energy to prepare healthier foods and eat them so that you are more likely to have these healthier options available for you. If cultivating the motivation for preparing and eating healthy foods has been problematic for you, this type of hypnosis focus can be incredibly helpful.

Using Hypnosis to Encourage Healthy Lifestyle Changes

In addition to helping you encourage yourself to eat healthier while discouraging yourself from eating unhealthy foods, you can also use hypnosis to help encourage you to make healthy lifestyle changes. This can support you with everything from exercising more frequently to picking up more active hobbies that support your wellbeing in general.

You may also use this to help you eliminate hobbies or experiences from your life that may encourage unhealthy dietary habits in the first place. For example, if you tend to binge eat when you are stressed out, you might use hypnosis to help you navigate stress more effectively so that you are less likely to binge eat when you are feeling stressed out. If you tend to eat when you are feeling emotional or bored, you can use hypnosis to help you change those behaviors, too.

Hypnosis can be used to change virtually any area of your life that motivates you to eat unhealthily or otherwise neglect self-care to the point where you are sabotaging yourself from healthy weight loss. It truly is an incredibly versatile practice that you can rely on that will help you with weight loss, as well as help you with creating a healthier lifestyle in general. With hypnosis, there are countless ways that you can improve the quality of your life, making it an incredibly helpful practice for you to rely on.

Weight loss via hypnosis will aid you in losing extra pounds when it's in a weight loss scheme that involves counseling, exercise, and diet.

Hypnosis is being in a state of your inner self, having good focus and absorption, such as being in a trance. This is commonly done with the aid of a professional hypnotherapist using oral recitations being repeated and mental pictures. During hypnosis, your focus is highly concentrated, and you're more reactive to suggestions, such as, behavioral changes that will aid you in losing weight.

Hypnosis is not a type of mind control, yet it is designed to alter your mind by shifting your feelings toward liking something that you might have hated before, such as exercise or eating a balanced diet. The same goes for quitting sugar or binge eating. Hypnosis identifies the root of the issues you may be dealing with and works by rectifying it accordingly. Given that it changes your thought pattern, you may also experience a much calmer and relaxed approach to everything you do.

Chapter 21. Why Is It Hard To Lose Weight?

Aside from hormonal and genetic factors, weight gain has a direct correlation to our negative emotions. Overindulgence and Overeating seem to be connected in our brains with specific events, relationships, feelings, and our thoughts have ascertained that in some cases, the food is serving a crucial reason, i.e., the usage of food inf comforting stress.

It appears everybody nowadays is attempting to lose weight. We are modified by our condition to look, dress, and even act in a specific way. Each time you get a magazine, turn on the TV or check out yourself, you are reminded of it. You start to hate your body losing control, disappointed, focused on, apprehensive, and now and again even discouraged.

If losing weight is tied in with eating fewer calories than your body needs and doing some activity to support your digestion, at that point, why are such a significant number of individuals as yet attempting to lose weight? Losing weight has to do with your considerations and convictions as much as it has to do with what you eat. Give me a chance to give you a model. You are staring at the TV, and an advertisement is shown demonstrating a chocolate cheddar cake that you can make utilizing just three fixings. You weren't hungry previously. However, since you have seen that cheddar cake, you might feel denied, and you need to eat. Your feelings are revealing to you that you have to eat, although your stomach isn't disclosing to you that you are hungry.

This is called emotional. It is our feelings that trigger our practices.

You may find that when you are feeling focused or depressed, you have this need to eat something since it solaces you somehow or another. The issue is that generally, it isn't healthy that you get for, and once you have done this a couple of times, it turns into a passionate stay, so every time that you experience pressure or grief, it triggers you to eat something.

Grapples keep you attached to convictions that you have about your life and yourself that prevent you from pushing ahead. You regularly compensate yourself with things that prevent you from losing weight. When you're utilizing nourishment to reward or repay yourself, you are managing stays.

Although the grapples that I am alluding to around passionate eating are not healthy ones, they can likewise be utilized intentionally to get a specific outcome.

Enthusiastic eating doesn't happen because you are physically hungry. It occurs because something triggers a craving for nourishment. You are either intuitively or deliberately covering a hidden, enthusiastic need.

Food has become the unconscious reflex when one is stressing out. Habits of the mind like this are exactly the reason for losing weight can be challenging a lot for people

Far down our unconscious minds, we have built rigid thoughts about behaviors that are not healthy. As a matter of fact, as time goes by, one might have developed the mind into believing that these behaviors that are not healthy are crucial, i.e., they are important for sustaining our good health. Suppose the mind is convinced these behaviors are much needed, change that is for the long runs is difficult. Motional eating or stress eating is just one instance out of several. There many unhealthy companies and associations we build that negatively influence our choice of food. Some usual associations that hinder weight loss involve:

- Consuming food is a convenient blanket, used for comforting one's self in times of depression or despair.

- When we eat, it brings a great distraction to us from feeling sad, worry or angry

- Excessive intake of sugary, fatty, or unhealthy foods is connected with party celebrations and other great times.

- Foods full of sugar or ones are a sort of reward or compensation.

- Overeating makes you reduce fearing that you won't be able to achieve losing weight

- Food can give one entertainment when one is feeling bored.

The fear of eating can assume control over your life. It expends your musings, depleting you of your vitality and self-discipline, making you separate and gorge. This will create more fear and make matters more regrettable. So how might you conquer your fear and different feelings around eating? You can transform the majority of your feelings around eating into another more beneficial relationship.

In all actuality, you have a soul. You should find it. It is that spot inside of you that is continually cherishing, forgiving and tranquil. It's a spot that speaks to your higher self, the genuine you, the sheltered, loved, and entire you. When you find this, the resentment, dissatisfaction, and stress that you are feeling about your weight will vanish.

Things never appear to happen as fast as we might want them to...perhaps your body isn't changing as quickly as you need. This may demoralize you giving you further reason to indulge. Comprehend that your body is a gift, and afterward, you will begin to contemplate it.

Quit harping on your stomach fat, your fat arms and butt, your enormous thighs that you hate and every one of the calories that you're taking in, and see all that your body is, all that your body can do and all that your body is doing right now. This new mindfulness will make love and acknowledgment for your body, such that you never had. You start to treasure it like the astounding gift that it is and center around, giving it wellbeing every day in each moment with each breath.

Begin concentrating on picking up wellbeing as opposed to losing weight, and you will be progressively happy, alive, and thankful. Find the delight of carrying on with a healthy life and feeding your soul consistently. Develop more love increasingly with your body and yourself, and this love will move and transform you from the inside out. When you tap into an option that is greater than you, you have the constant motivation, which is far more dominant than any battle of the mind or feelings. Tolerating and adoring your body precisely as it is correct presently is the thing that sends the mending vibrations that will quiet your mind and transform your body from the inside out.

When you figure out how to love and acknowledge your body, you are in arrangement with your higher self....that adoring and inviting self.

Grasp what your identity is and not who you think you are or ought to be. Understand the endeavors that you make are seeds. Try not to see the majority of your efforts to lose weight as disappointments, consider them to be seeds you are planting towards progress.

Pardon yourself. Try not to thrash yourself, regardless of how frequently you think you've fizzled, irrespective of what you resemble at this moment and irrespective of how often you need that new beginning. Pardon yourself!

Chapter 22. How Can Hypnosis Help You Lose Weight?

The very commencement of using hypnosis for weight loss is by identifying the reason for your not achieving goals. How effective is this? Quintessentially, a hypnotherapist will ask you question in line with your weight loss, i.e., questions which revolves around your eating and exercise habits.

The coalition of this information helps recognize what you might need help working on. You would after that be put be through induction, a process where the mind and body relaxes and enter into a state of hypnosis. During hypnosis, your mind is highly opened. You've neglected your critical, conscious mind – and the hypnotherapist can speak straightly to your unconscious thoughts. In hypnosis, the hypnotherapist will give you positive suggestions, affirmations and may ask you to imagine changes.

Here are the positive suggestions for weight loss hypnosis:

Enhancing Confidence. Positive suggestions will improve your feelings of confidence via encouraging or soothing language.

Envisaging Success. In hypnosis, you may be asked to envisage attaining your weight loss targets and imagine the way it makes you feel.

Restructuring Your Inner Voice. Hypnosis can help your control your inner voice who "wouldn't want" to quit unhealthy food habits and turn it into support in your weight loss journey, which's fast with positive suggestions and is more rational.

Selecting the Unconscious. During the hypnotic state, you can start to recognize the unconscious patterns that birth unhealthy eating. In order words, you can become more observant of our choices for making unhealthy food, quantity control, and establishing more useful and conscious strategies for making choices.

Complete subdue of fear. Hypnotic suggestions can aid in suppressing your fear of not attaining weight loss goals. Fear is a fundamental reason people shy away from starting in the first place.

Recognizing and Restructuring Habit Patterns. During hypnosis, you can always observe and explore ways you used eating in turning off these automatic responses. Through regular continuity of positive affirmations, we can start slowing and eventually completely remove automatic, unconscious thinking.

Building New Coping Techniques. Through hypnosis, you can create a healthier medium of coping with stress, emotions, and relationships. For instance, you might be asked to imagine a stressful condition and then picture yourself responding with healthy snacks.

Practicing Healthy Eating. While in hypnosis, you may be asked to practice making healthy eating choices, i.e., being good with taking food home at a restaurant. This enhances these healthy choices to become more automatic. The practice is also helpful and amply useful in controlling cravings.

Making Good and Useful Food Choices. Of course, you possibly may desire and love unhealthy foods, but hypnosis can help you grow a taste or preference for healthier choices, as well as control the portion sizes of your choice.

Increase in Unconscious Signals. Through repeated pattern, you may have learned to recognize and pin-point indicators your body sends when you feel full. Hypnotherapy helps to notice these signals.

For sure, not all suggestions might work for you. Your hypnotherapy scheme, either you are working with a hypnotherapist or via self-hypnosis –will involve suggestions important to your relationship with food. For instance, Janet (from those as mentioned earlier) might work on instructing the unconscious of delaying its automatic responses, as well as giving the unconscious new, more helpful ways to handle stress. Communicating with a licensed hypnotherapist can help you discover your strategy to be your exact needs.

While in a hypnotic state, your mind is much more susceptible to suggestions. As a matter of fact, a study has revealed that some dramatic changes take place in your brain during hypnosis, which permits you to learn without critical thought about the information you're receiving.

In other words, you are separated from the critical mind. Hence, when you receive hypnotic suggestions, the critical consciousness of the mind doesn't come into play what you hear. That, in conclusion, is how hypnosis can help you break through the barriers that hinder you from losing weight. With repetition being a critical process for success, much reason most hypnotherapists send you home with reference to self-hypnosis recordings after the first visit. The limitation in your mind is tough, only through continuous repeated work will you satisfactorily untangle and reshape the convictions.

Though, listening to repeated affirmations and positive suggestions as to healthy eating is a first step in the weight loss trip. You're instructing your mind to think in a different way, but these convictions can help you.

Manage Cravings

What if you could withdraw from your cravings? Seclude them and send them away? Some weight loss hypnosis strategies assist you in doing this. For instance, you might be asked to imagine sending away your lustful appetite (cravings). Suggestions can help reshape a lustful appetite, and learn to control them efficiently.

Anticipate Success

Anticipation births reality. When we have anticipation for success, we are more likely to take the necessary steps to reach that goal. Weight loss hypnotherapy can implant in you the seed of success in your mind, which can be a potent unconscious influencer to keep you on track.

Practice Positivity

Weight loss is often destroyed by negativity. There are foods you can't eat. Unhealthy foods are detrimental to you. Hypnotherapy strengthens us to reshape these suggestions with a more positive light. It's not a denial of oneself. It's just refraining yourself from what your body doesn't need.

Options for Hypnosis to Lose Weight

Are you really ready to kick start your weight loss journey? To start off, there are several options. Visiting a professional hypnotherapist physically for a session or fix up a virtual conference with a hypnotherapist will be fine. Recorded hypnosis or self-hypnosis is another option. All method as regards hypnosis has shown promising result for weight loss.

One-on-One Hypnosis - A hypnotherapist can assist you in recognizing the unconscious limitations that are holding your bond. Additionally, a hypnotherapist sees you through in those sessions to resolve the limitations. These are done in offices or better done via video conferencing.

Guided Hypnosis: A guided hypnosis record can aid you to get quickly started and learn hypnosis mechanisms at your residence or on the go. More importantly, these are records from certified hypnotherapists that walk you through induction and then give positive suggestion through the recording.

Self-Hypnosis; engaging in self-hypnosis, individuals take on the responsibility of hypnotherapists, making use of a memorized script to lure them into hypnosis and, after that, deliver positive suggestions. Get lose from every habit and attain your weight loss targets.

Shut your eyes, visualize your food cravings going off, imagine a day of eating only what's best for you. Imagine hypnosis eventually helping you lose weight- because the news is; it does. Here are ten hypnotic suggestions to try straight away.

Several people have not come to the knowledge and recognition that adding trance to your weight loss scheme can help lose more weight and keep it off farther.

Hypnosis precedes calorie counting by a few centuries, but attention hasn't been given to the long-aged techniques, not embracing completely as an effective strategy of weight loss. Very recently, there has been a scant scientific proof to support the legitimate resolutions of respected hypnotherapists,

Even after the convincing and compelling mid-nineties evaluations of 18 hypnotic types of research revealed that psychotherapy clients who learned self-hypnosis lost double as much weight as those who didn't. Hypnotherapy, therefore, has been a well-kept weight loss mystery.

Until hypnosis has happily forced you or someone you know to buy a new, smaller wardrobe, it may be quite difficult to be convinced that this mind-over technique could help you get a handle on eating.

Chapter 23. Hypnosis To Eliminate Cravings And For Portion Control

Whether you wish to shed many pounds or maintain a healthy weight, proper portion consumption is as necessary as the consumption of appropriate foods. The rate of obesity among youngsters and adults has increased partly owing to the increase in restaurant portions.

A portion is the total quantity of food that you eat in one sitting. A serving size is the suggested quantity of one particular food. For instance, the amount of steak you eat for dinner maybe a portion; however, three ounces of steak, maybe a serving. Controlling serving sizes helps with portion control.

Health Benefits of Portion Control

Serious health problems are caused by overeating. For example, type 2 diabetes, weight problems, high blood pressure, and many more. Therefore, when you are looking to lead a healthy lifestyle, portion control should be a significant priority.

Fullness and Weight Management

Feeling satiable, or having a sense of fullness, will affect the quantity you eat and the way you usually eat. According to the British Nutrition Foundation, eating smaller portions slowly increases the feeling of satiety after a meal.

Eating smaller parts also permits your body to use the food you eat right away for energy, rather than storing the excess as fat. Losing weight is not as straightforward as solely controlling your portion sizes; however, once you learn to observe the quantity of food you eat, you will begin to apply conscious intake, which might assist you in making healthier food decisions.

When you eat too quickly, you do not notice your stomach's cues that it is full. Eat slowly and listen to hunger cues to enhance feelings of fullness and, ultimately, consume less food.

Improved Digestion

Considerably larger portion sizes contribute to an upset stomach and discomfort (caused by a distended stomach pushing down on your other organs). Your gastrointestinal system functions best when it is not full of food. Managing portions can help to get rid of cramping and bloating after eating. You furthermore may run the danger of getting pyrosis, as a result of having a full abdomen will push hydrochloric acid back into your digestive tract.

Money Savings

Eating smaller parts may lead to monetary benefits, mainly when eating out. In addition to eating controlled serving sizes, you do not have to purchase as many groceries. Measuring serving proportions can make the box of cereal and packet of nuts last longer than eating straight out of the container.

Take, for instance, the method to apply portion management at restaurants is to order kid-sized meals, that are typically cheaper than adult meals and closer to the right serving size you ought to be eating.

Adult portion sizes at restaurants will equal two, three, or even more servings. Therefore, immediately the food arrives at your table, request for a takeaway container and put away half of your food from the plate.

Take your food home, and this way, you will have two meals for the worth of one.

How to Control Portions Using Hypnosis

Hypnosis can take you into a deeply relaxed state and quickly train your mind to understand when to do away with excess food instinctively, and allow your digestion to be lighter, and more comfortable. You may discover the pleasure of being in tune with what your own body requires nourishment. Hypnosis will re-educate your instincts to regulate hunger pangs. As you relax and repeatedly listen to powerful hypnotic suggestions that are going to be absorbed by your mind; you may quickly begin to note that:

- Your mind is no longer engrossed in food
- Your abdomen and gut feel lighter
- You now do not feel uncontrollable hunger pangs at 'non-meal' times
- You naturally forget to have food between meals
- You begin to enjoy a healthier lifestyle

There is a somewhat simple self-hypnosis process for helping you control your appetite and portions. In a shell, you are immersing yourself into a psychological state and picture a dial, or a flip switch of some type that is symbolic of your craving and your real hunger. Then you repeatedly apply to develop a true sense of control, then you employ it out of the hypnotic state and when confronted with those things and circumstances to curb the perceived hunger and control your appetite.

Step 1: Get yourself into a comfortable position and one where you will remain undisturbed for the period of this exercise. Ascertain your feet are flat on the ground and hands not touching. Then once you are in position, calm yourself.

You can do that by using hypnosis tapes; they are basic processes to assist you in opening the door of your mind.

Step 2: You may prefer to deepen your hypnotic state. The best and most straightforward is imagining yourself in your favorite place and relaxing your body bit by bit. Keep focused on the session at hand (that is, watch out not to drift off) then go to the third step.

Step 3: Take a picture of a dial, a lever, or a flippy switch of some kind that is on a box or mounted on a wall of some sort-let it fully controls your mind's eye. Notice the colors, the materials that it is created out of, and the way it indicates 0-10 to mark the variable degrees of your real hunger.

Notice wherever it is indicating currently let it show you how hungry you are. Remember when last you ate, what you ate, whether or not the hunger is genuine, or merely reacting to a recent bout of gluttony and wanting to gratify that sensation!

Once you have established the dial, where it is set, and trusting that the reading is correct, then go to the subsequent step.

Step 4: Flip the dial down a peg and notice the effects taking place within you. Study your feedback and ascertain that it feels like you are moving your appetite with the dial. The more you believe you are affecting your appetite with the dial, the more practical its application in those real-life situations.

Practice turning it down even lower and start recognizing how you use your mind to change your perceived appetite utilizing a method that is healthy and helps keep you alert when you encounter circumstances with plenty of food supply. Tell yourself that the more you observe this, the better control you gain over your appetite.

You might even create a strong affirmation that accompanies this dial "I am in control of my eating" is one such straightforward statement. Word it as you wish and make sure it is one thing that resonates well with you. Once you have repeated the meaningful affirmations to yourself several times with conviction, proceed to the next step.

Step 5: Visualize yourself during a future scenario, where there is going to be constant temptation to continue eating although you are full, or to consume an excessive amount. See the sights of that place, take a mental note of the other people there, notice the smells, hear the sounds. Become increasingly aware of how you are feeling in this place. Get the most definition and clarity possible, then notice that once the temptation presents itself, you turn down the dial on your craving. You realize that you are not hungry to eat anymore, then repeat your positive affirmations to yourself a few more times to strengthen it.

Run through this future state of affairs severally on loop to make sure your mind is mentally rehearsed about your plan to respond.

Step 6: Twitch your little finger and toes, then open your eyes and proceed to observe your skills in real-life and spot how much control you have.

Chapter 24. Hypnotherapy for Weight Loss

The subconscious mind has immense control over the actions of our bodies. And over our subconscious mind, we have great control. But are we sure of how to use it? Will we understand our minds enough to handle it correctly and take advantage of this advantage for us? We may ask someone to use it for us if we do not.

The conscious mind can drive an idea by repetitive thoughts into the subconscious mind. In a certain amount of time, the idea is set such that the subconscious mind pushes the body to act on the idea.

This is the basic information on which this theory is based. A hypnosis specialist will also aid us if we can not do this ourselves (fix an idea into the subconscious). Of course, it's much easier to say than to do.

Firstly, since weight loss hypnotherapy can sound like a good idea, but it can make the difference between success and failure to find the right therapist. Seek to get positive advice from close friends or experts in the area.

Secondly, because old habits die pretty hard, and you can only hope that you are close to the desired results after several weeks or even months of intensive treatment.

Thirdly, that at the beginning of your new body, you will feel very nervous, and you will wake up to ideas "plants" inside your mind that get stronger and stronger. This could take some time to get used to.

In all of this, we can conclude that although weight loss hypnotherapy can seem a pretty easy process before you go into the theory, there are a few things to consider. For one, I don't want anyone to worry about my subconscious mind.

Reasons Why Hypnotherapy for Weight Loss Works

For too many people, weight loss is the ultimate (and unattainable) target. Dozens of products are available on the fitness market-supplements, dietary plans, workout programs, and even "miracle" solutions. Most of these goods will not achieve the desired outcome since weight loss is a complex operation.

Hypnosis of weight loss is one viable alternative. In comparison to other eating plans and drugs, it provides a comprehensive solution. Hypnotherapy discusses the physiological causes of overweight persistence and thus produces positive outcomes.

Good Encouragement

All the limitations are traditional weight loss. You'll learn what foods to avoid, what bad habits to give up, and how to track your progress constantly. In these cases, constructive energy would be absent.

Hypnosis in weight loss focuses on the positive. It shifts underlying patterns of thought. Instead of thinking that burgers will make you fat, you will discover that carrots will improve your health and provide important vitamins to your body.

Positive hypnotic advice teaches you how to love your body and enjoy good health. It is much easier to maintain the system if you are happy and positive about it.

Coping with Stress

Will you want to eat more any time you are tired, nervous, lonely, or depressed? If so, you're unhealthy with food and relying on the wrong mechanism of coping.

Hypnosis allows you to uncover the triggers for stress, anxiety, and even self-pity. These emotional factors overtake you and form your relationship with food.

Auto-consciousness allows you to escape circumstances that make you feel bad. Furthermore, you learn how to cope without turning to food. A healthier coping strategy is always enough to lose weight and lead to a healthy lifestyle.

Benefits of Hypnotherapy for Weight Loss

The food industry is a billion-dollar industry and shows no sign of a slowdown. How many diets have you just tried to boom to the biscuit tin?? Who doesn't realize that less and more is the secret to weight loss? Certainly, we do not lack 'details.' So, why the battle? I will let you in the secret because when it comes to making permanent changes, your conscious mind (which is your willpower) is tight, your unconscious mind is here the true powerhouse. When you remember all of the above, and it has not changed yet, then it's doubtful you'll change it either, so it might be time to try weight loss hypnotherapy.

- Emotional eating
- Eat when you're not hungry
- Compulsive eating (wondering why you are doing this but can't stop)
- The cycle of compulsion - guilt - punishment.

Your unconscious biases (which you actually don't know about, but which are revealed during hypnotherapy for weight loss) motivate your food relationship. As youngsters, we may have been told "to finish everything on our plates," and these old messages can still be played. Or maybe we grew up with a mother who troubled her weight, or maybe we saw food as "love," and we comforted ourselves and "love" today when we felt weak, depressed, anxious, or lonely.

It's not about diets, it's about feelings, and how you 'use' food to change them, this is why weight loss hypnotherapy works so well for feelings and thought patterns. For women, food is also their choice of medicines. It might well be time to dive and try hypnotherapy to lose weight for true independence and an improved, safe link to food and exercise for life.

Is Hypnotherapy The Answer For Weight Loss

For all the demands modern lives impose on individuals, weight loss can be difficult to achieve. It is no wonder that men, women, and even children are feeding on the road more and more. The standard Western diet known as S.A.D. is high in sugar, fat and simple carbohydrates, and of course, chemical additives. This diet makes people obese and triggers a diabetes epidemic and other associated diseases. In fact, people are traveling less. The average citizen is busy and exhausted, but not enough physically.

Stress is a significant factor in poor lifestyle choices and can lead to bad habits. Individuals who have gained weight are mindful of what they are doing, but it is difficult to find encouragement if the burden keeps piling. We just want someone else to stay in their bodies (with a healthy diet and workout habits) for a little while to help push things in the right direction. Hypnosis will help here. The new person who resides inside his body maybe them!

Hypnosis operates at a subconscious level by giving the subconscious mind clear suggestions. Good ideas to encourage weight loss research at an unconscious level in order to build new attitudes, principles, and traditional thought so that consumers can make healthy decisions. Hypnosis encourages a positive lifestyle transition leading to the reduction of body weight. It's so good, therefore. Diets have shown long-term ineffectiveness while modifying the diet and maintaining habits leads to positive results in weight loss.

Hypnosis strategies for weight loss typically include reinforcement of motivation and confidence building phrases as well as clear instructions for a healthy lifestyle. Hypnosis exercises often typically use visualization techniques to help the client "see" his target weight and "feel" what it looks like. This makes them successful. If a person can think he can lose weight, he can. Sadly, many people have attempted many diets and failed, thus losing their self-confidence and desire to take away their weight. Weight loss hypnosis focuses on how people feel when they lose weight, their desire to do so, and on the process of adopting a new, healthier lifestyle.

Hypnosis deals with multiple individuals differently. Some people respond to suggestions very easily and adjust them consistently for a long time, resulting in faster weight loss. Some, however, take longer and longer sessions to retrain the subconscious mind and alter their perceptions about themselves, what they are willing to do, and what they really want to do. To change their lifestyle successfully, people really want to do it.

Persons with hypnosis to lose weight will find that it offers a number of potential health benefits that are not specifically linked to weight loss. Hypnosis soothes the mind, nerves, and the entire body. It relieves anxiety and reduces tension. The recommendations include confidence and self-esteem that help every aspect of customer's lives. People who use hypnosis for a particular purpose also consider several unintended advantages. The gentleness of the approach also offers a healthy, supportive, and simple way to support a child or teenager with excessive weight.

Chapter 25. Step By Step Guide To Hypnotherapy For Weight Loss

Hypnotherapy is the use of hypnosis in the care of patients who have discomfort or difficulties inside their minds. Those using hypnotherapy claim patients experiencing a trance have higher chances to listen to the advice they are being given.

Shut your eyes, breathe, relax. Visualize yourself resisting the lure to overindulge. Imagine you not having cravings for unhealthy foods. Envisage that you don't need to comfort your appetite with food. If weight loss has been that easy, you might have the thought that if only you could "shut up" your unhealthy cravings. Anyway, that's the concept of hypnosis for weight loss. Harnessing hypnotherapy, those who want to lose weight are empowered to improve on the automatic thoughts that facilitate food cravings.

But, if you can afford to undergo a series of hypnotherapy sessions with a specialist, you may do so. This is ideal as you will work with a professional who can guide you through the treatment and will also provide you valuable advice on nutrition and exercises.

Clinical Hypnotherapy

In your first session, the therapist will commonly start by explaining to you the type of hypnotherapy he or she is using. Then you will discuss your personal goals so the therapist can better understand your motivations.

The formal session will start with your therapist, speaking in a gentle and soothing voice. This will aid you in relaxing and feeling safe during the entire therapy.

Once your mind is more receptive, the therapist will start suggesting ways that can help you modify your exercise or eating habits as well as other ways to help you reach your weight loss goals.

Specific words or repetition of specific phrases can help you at this stage. The therapist may also help you in visualizing the body image you want, which is one effective technique in hypnotherapy.

To end the session, the therapist will bring you out from the hypnotic stage, and you will start to be more alert. Your personal goals will influence the duration of the hypnotherapy sessions, as well as the number of total sessions that you may need. Most people begin to see results in as few as two to four sessions.

DIY Hypnotherapy

If you are not comfortable working with a professional hypnotherapist or you just can't afford the sessions, you can choose to perform self-hypnosis. While this is not as effective as the sessions under a professional, you can still try it and see if it can help you with your weight loss goals.

Here are the steps if you wish to practice self-hypnosis:

Believe in the power of hypnotism. Remember, this alternative treatment requires the person to be open and willing. It will not work for you if your mind is already set against it.

Find a comfortable and quiet room to practice hypnotherapy. Ideally, you must seek a place or room that is free from noise and where no one can disturb you. Wear loose clothes and set relaxing music to help in setting up the mood.

Find a focal point. Choose an object in a room that you can focus on. Use your concentration on this object so you can start clearing your mind of all thoughts.

Breathe deeply. Start with five deep breaths, inhaling through your nose and exhaling through your mouth.

Close your eyes. Think about your eyelids becoming heavy and just let them close slowly.

Imagine that all stress and tension are coming out of your body. Let this feeling move down from your head, to your shoulders, to your chest, to your arms, to your stomach, to your legs, and finally to your feet.

Clear your mind. When you are totally relaxed, your mind must be clear, and you can initiate the process of self-hypnotism.

Visualize a pendulum. In your mind, picture a moving pendulum. The movement of the pendulum is popular imagery used in hypnotism to encourage focus.

Start visualizing your ideal body image and size. This should help you instill in your subconscious the importance of a healthy diet and exercise. Suggest to yourself to avoid unhealthy food and start exercising regularly. You can use a particular mantra such as "I will exercise at least three times a week. Unhealthy food will make me sick."

Wake up. Once you have achieved what you want during hypnosis, you must wake yourself. Start by counting back from one to 10, and wake up when you reach 10.

Remember, a healthy diet doesn't mean that you have to reduce your food intake significantly. Just reduce your intake of food that is not healthy for you. Never hypnotize yourself out of eating. Just suggest to yourself to eat less of the food that you know is just making you fat.

Chapter 26. Hypnosis For Food And Sugar Addiction

Looking good and being healthy are not only the personal motives of most of us, but it is also our responsibility to take care of the bodies we have been blessed with. If we are not going to take care of our health, what we eat, how much we weigh, and how good we look, then who will? I have encountered people who are in a desperate state for wanting to look slim and fit, but their actions speak otherwise. They not only consume tonnes of junk foods but also refrain from doing any sort of exercise. What you need is a motivated set up of the mind, and then the action required in achieving the desired results would not be boring. In fact, it would be "inspired action." Self-hypnosis blesses you with this motivation for inspired action, due to which you would not feel bored or lazy while taking action to achieve your goals. This part is a self-hypnosis guide for weight loss and thereby solution to your associated problems of obesity, Diabetes Mellitus, heart diseases, and high blood pressure.

Recording your power-script:

1. Choose a serene and calm place for recording your power script. Voice of some person or any sort of noise can interfere with the recordings. Natural sounds like the chirping of birds or flowing of water in the background (in case you choose a riverside for recordings) are not only acceptable but also lay a calming effect on you while you are listening to the recording during hypnosis. You may ask the question, "Isn't the voice of any person (like a family member) in the background

a natural sound?" It surely is, but what if there is a negative talk going on in the background, I am pretty sure you won't like yourself to program negative thoughts into your subconscious mind. So, it is better to choose a calm, natural, and noise-free place for recordings.

2. Use your audio recording device to record the power-script, which is mentioned below.

Getting ready for self-hypnosis:

3. Bring the audio device to the place where you intend to go for self-hypnosis. The place should also be a calm one, like your bedroom or study room.

4. Plugin the earphones into the device and insert them into your ears. You can use headphones as well in case these are not heavy. Using better quality ear/headphones is recommended.

5. You should preferably sit in a chair that is comfortable for this task. It should not be too warm and cozy or cold (like steel chairs). It should be absolutely perfect for sitting. Lying on the bed can make you feel sleepy, especially when you go for the task at night time or after some heavy physical work. So, avoid using bed and make sure to use a comfortable chair for the task.

6. After adjusting yourself in the chair, inserting earphones in ears, and just before you are going to press the play button of your recording device, do to yourself pre-induction self-talk that you will surely undergo hypnosis by yourself and will be benefited by the same.

7 Now, press the play button of the audio device and close your eyes. The script plays:

THE SCRIPT:

Progressive relaxation:

"I'm going to adjust my body so that I am in a comfortable position.

I am noticing all spots in my body where I am carrying the tension of the day. I am now making the decision to let go of that tension.

One by one, I am moving my legs, my thighs, my buttocks, my back, my chest, my arms, my hands, my shoulders, and my head till I feel every part is at ease and not tense.

......I am now closing my eyes......

I am concentrating on my breathing, inhaling, and exhaling the fresh air. I am feeling my nose, chest muscles, abdomen, chest muscles again, and finally, my mouth as they are being filled with air from inspiration to expiration.

......I am feeling relaxed with each breath I take......

Now I am tensing my legs and feet tightly and then releasing the tension. I am doing it again for the second time. I can feel my legs and feet muscles get relaxed.

Now I am tensing my thighs and then releasing the tension. I am doing it again for the second time. I can feel the muscles of my thighs getting relaxed.

Now I am tensing my buttocks and then releasing the tension. I am doing it again for the second time. I can feel the muscles of my buttocks getting relaxed.

Now I am tensing my back and then releasing the tension. I am doing it again for the second time. I can feel the muscles of my back getting relaxed.

Now I am tensing my abdomen and then releasing the tension. I am doing it again for the second time. I can feel the muscles of my abdomen getting relaxed.

Now I am tensing my chest and then releasing the tension. I am doing it again for the second time. I can feel the muscles of my chest getting relaxed.

Now I am tensing my shoulders and then releasing the tension. I am doing it again for the second time. I can feel the muscles of my shoulders getting relaxed.

Now I am tensing my arms, forearms, and hands, and then releasing the tension. I am doing it again for the second time. I can feel the muscles of my arms, forearms, and hands getting relaxed.

Now I am tensing my neck and then releasing the tension. I am doing it again for the second time. I can feel the muscles of my neck getting relaxed.

Now I am tensing my face and scalp and then releasing the tension. I am doing it again for the second time. I can feel the muscles of my face and scalp getting relaxed.

.....Since all my muscles are relaxed, I am going to fill my body parts with a special pleasing sensation......

With one breath I take in, I am imagining that the breath is moving to my right buttock, thigh, and leg. With the exhalation, I am feeling a special relaxing sensation in my right buttock, thigh, and leg.

With one breath I take in, I am imagining that the breath is moving to my left buttock, thigh, and leg. With an exhalation, I am feeling a special relaxing sensation in my left buttock, thigh, and leg.

With one breath I take in, I am imagining that the breath is moving to my lower back and abdomen. With an exhalation, I am feeling a special relaxing sensation in my lower back and abdomen.

With one breath I take in, I am imagining that the breath is moving to my upper back and chest. With an exhalation, I am feeling a special relaxing sensation in my upper back and chest.

With one breath I take in, I am imagining that the breath is moving from my neck, through shoulders to both my arms, forearms, and hands. With an exhalation, I am feeling a special relaxing sensation in my neck, shoulders, arms, forearms, and hands.

With one breath I take in, I am imagining that the breath is moving through my nose to my forehead, to my scalp, and then through my face back into the air through my mouth. With an exhalation, I am feeling a special relaxing sensation in my forehead, scalp, face, and mouth.

......I am feeling super relaxed, calm, enjoying this special experience, and I am now ready for the process of visualization."

Visualization

[Record the following emotionalized visualization and while recording as well as while you are playing the script, try to get a real feeling of what you are visualizing]

"I am enjoying a party where everyone who knew me before is staring at me. I will try to figure out why they are doing so. Meanwhile, while having a conversation with one of my friends, I see a gorgeous person in the large mirror that is placed nearby. Who is this slim, trim, well-dressed person? I can't wait to go close to the mirror and figure out if it really is me. Is this the reason why everyone is looking at me with a 'look'

141

that reveals that they are highly impressed with my slim and attractive personality? Or are their eyes trying to figure out how I lost so much weight? Well, this old friend of mine shakes my hand and says, "You look awesome. How come do you manage to maintain such a slim shape of your body?" I can feel the joy and the happiness of this comment as well as the confidence which this new slim look is blessing me.

.....Now, I am ready to accept the hypnotic suggestions for my own benefit."

Hypnotic suggestions

I am in love with my slim and toned body.

My body is healthier, slimmer, and stronger than before.

I love feeling light and free.

I am at my perfect weight, healthy and slim.

I am getting slimmer and healthy every day.

I am eating only healthy and nutritious foods.

I love eating a balanced diet with more fresh fruits and salads.

I enjoy drinking a lot of water every day.

I am taking all the actions I need to maintain my weight.

I like waking up early in the morning and enjoying the fresh air while running.

I like to exercise as every drop of sweat is making me realize that my weight is becoming less.

I enjoy exercising, and my fitness schedule is giving me fantastic results.

I am blessed with a healthy physique and 100% working metabolism

I am in love with working out hard and pushing my limits.

I am in love with working out because it is making me feel slimmer and healthier every minute.

I am feeling satisfied with my healthy thoughts, balanced diet, and fruitful exercise.

My body is naturally getting slimmer and healthier.

I am wearing the clothes of my own choice with perfect fitting.

I have a confident and healthy personality.

I am blessed with the 'slim and healthy shape' of my body, and I am maintaining this shape.

Waking up from the hypnotic state

I am now waking up from the state of hypnosis.

I am waking up to take positive action towards updating my newly imagined version of myself.

I am now fully programmed with the power-script for weight loss.

I am waking up to see how motivated I am.

I am feeling fresh and positive.

I am opening my eyes now

Chapter 27. Conditions For Hypnosis To Work Out

Although hypnosis itself cannot be accurately predicted, clinical experience and laboratory experiments at institutions such as Harvard and Stanford suggest that those who are most susceptible to hypnosis tend to share certain characteristics. As already mentioned, virtually everyone can benefit from hypnosis. However, if you have most of these characteristics, studies have shown that you may be easier to hypnotize than others. Here are some of the criteria for hypnosis:

- Motivation

The motivation is at the top of the list. If you don't want to be hypnotized, you won't. If you are strong enough to change something, the chance is to be able to hypnotize yourself. But such motives must come from within. You need to want to change yourself, not because other people think you should, but because it's what you need at the moment.

- Optimism

Top people tend not to be skeptics if you take a continuum of hypnosis from low to high. This doesn't mean you can't hypnotize yourself if you're skeptical now. However, we hope that by the end of this topic, your skepticism will be alleviated somewhat so that you can experience hypnosis more easily. It turns out that most hypnotic people are likely to have a hopeful and optimistic view of life. To them, the bottle is not half empty but half full.

- Defending

The people most susceptible to hypnosis are usually lawyers. This is an extension of buoyancy, trust, and hope reflected in their optimism. Whether it's something new in medicine, politics, art, or something that interests them, they are keen to spread the word. An opposite is a person who is very cognitive and very scientific in her evaluation. This individual demand evidence wants to read half a dozen books and scrutinizes the subject before committing himself. This attitude of the brain is not wrong. It simply means that such reality-oriented individuals must stay longer in hypnosis to get results.

- Concentration

An important feature of hypnosis is increased concentration. Hypnosis deepens your concentration, but you need it to achieve this condition. The more distracting a person is, the more he responds if he tries to hypnotize himself or is hypnotized by others. He also has to use this method more often to make a profit. Meanwhile, most people at least sometimes have a deep focus. Go to the room when they are reading and call their name. You can't get the answer. Those people can't hear your voice because they are too concentrated. We find no significant evidence difference between vigorous situation and self-hypnosis itself.

- Acceptability

Many people are afraid to be hypnotized so as not to be absorbed in the will of others. This may be called Svengali syndrome. A mysterious stranger with a black cloak and flint's eyes seizes the soul of a naked girl while bending her will to adapt to an embarrassing wish. People who are prone to hypnosis have normal or good intelligence and a core of beliefs and firm attitudes that are fundamental to life. An example of such a person is someone with a well-trained religious education that embraces new ideas. He is hard to be fooled. He is sensitive to wise suggestions. Of course, the receptivity level differs from person to person. The receptivity for new ideas is one of the determinants of how easily you can get hypnosis. On a scale of 0-5 (0 is a person impervious to hypnosis), the majority of the population falls in the middle, for example, in the range 2 to 3. However, rest assured that your level of susceptibility to hypnosis is not included in the five-point scale. At the age of two or three, hypnosis should be repeated more often. However, being at the top of the scale has both disadvantages and benefits.

- Imagination

Scientists at the Hypnosis Institute at Stanford University School of Psychology have been studying the hypnotic differences between individuals for nearly two decades. This is a project supported by the National Mental Health Institute and the Air Force Office of Scientific Laboratory. An organization that does not tend to fund trivial efforts. Dr. Josephine R. Hilgard, a clinical professor of psychiatry at Stanford University, reported on the study: For some reason, people who have been imaginatively active as a child can have hypnosis. The theory states that the imagination and ability to participate in adventures that emerged early in life remained alive and functional through continued use. Among university students, reading, drama, creativity, childhood imagination, religion, sensory, and thirst for adventure were activities identified as hypnosis. Hypnosis is deeply involved in one or more imaginary areas (reading novels, listening to music, experiencing the aesthetic of nature, adventuring the body and mind) can do. "

Dr. Hilgard found that the student in major of humanities is most susceptible to hypnosis, the majors of social sciences are comparatively less, and students of natural sciences and engineering are not much hypnotized. The experience and research of other employees in this area tend to corroborate Stanford University results. According to Dr. Lewis R. Wolberg, a 40-year authority in the field: people with the ability to enjoy sensory stimulations and can adapt themselves to different roles have more tendency to be hypnotic than others.

Dr. Hilgard's lab was the most vulnerable to those who had fictitious friends in childhood and could read, adventure, and be immersed in nature. Suspicious, withdrawn, and hostile people have discovered that they tend to resist hypnosis. "Few people appreciate all of the above criteria. You don't even have to show improvement in all areas. You can make up for what's not present in another category. Defined these criteria, Hypnosis still needs a great deal of research, and the academic and medical community has accepted it as a subject worthy of serious investigation. A lot of eye-widening results are drawn from the research.

Chapter 28. Meditation For Weight Loss

Find a place to sit or lie down that is peaceful for complete relaxation, then breathe and pay attention. Notice as the air tides in through your nostrils and how your belly buzzes to the maximum and gently falls back to your spine as you breathe out. Allow gravity to hold you securely in place. Breathe as naturally as you can. Do not force your breathing and take notice if your breath is quick or slow and steady.

As you breathe in, accept gratitude and let warmth fill your lungs. Think of the things you are grateful for. Think of something that makes you feel happy and peaceful. Say to yourself, "I am thankful to be alive. I am secure and safe. I am confident and pure." Pay attention to your heart now. As you say these words to yourself, feel them deep within you. Give these statements positive energy and feed them with love. "I love myself; I can do anything I put my mind to. I trust that my brain, body, and soul are capable of providing me with what I desire most in life."

Breathe in now and fill your mind and soul with love and warmth. Imagine as you breathe in that there is a radiant light that fills your lungs before rapidly escaping your body. This light gives your patience, it gives you strength, and it provides you with the ambition and motivation to tackle the barriers that stand in your way. Breathe out naturally and notice as your body becomes heavier. With every breath that flows out, let go of negative thoughts; push those thoughts aside. You are good enough. You can do this. You are loved. You are special. Breathe out and release all of the tension that holds you back now. What other people believe and what you think are two different things. Say this now, "I believe in myself."

Count your breaths now. As you breathe in, breathe with your belly and count. One, two, three, four, and five. When you let go of this breath, make sure it is steady and slow. Breathe out, two, three, four, five. You are accepting this positive light to vibrate through your entire being. You are letting go of all the negativity that holds you back. Breathe in one, two, three, four. Breathe out one, two, three, four. And inhale for one, "I am happy," two, "I am strong," three, "I am kind," four, "I am brave," five, "I am driven to succeed." Breathe out now. You are counting your breath from one to five slow and steady. Positivity embraces you now; you feel light and in complete control. Nothing can disturb you; nothing can bring you down; you are perfect the way you are. Repeat this step until you are ready to watch your thoughts flow in and out.

Bring focus to your inner thoughts now. What pops into your mind? If you have any bad thoughts, let them be there as long as they want to be without judging them. Watch them, and then let them go. With every in-breath, notice your thoughts pop in without judgment. These thoughts are neither positive nor negative. When you breathe out, just let go of all hostility and anger you might be holding. Let it escape into the universe and breathe in, one, two, three, four, five; you are accepting all honesty and trust within yourself that you can make it through anything. "I am resilient. I am beautiful. I am a leader."

If you notice any negative thoughts, just see them and replace them with positive, self-loving thoughts.

Breaking Barriers

Ensure that you are presently in the place where you are completely comfortable and will not be disturbed for at least thirty minutes. Have the room you are inset to a comforting temperature and make sure that the lights are low. Adjust your body so that your shoulders are relaxed, your arms are lying on either side of you, and your palms are facing the ceiling. You want to become as comfortable and relaxed as you can so that your focus is not on your body but on the meditation. Gently close your eyes and take a deep breath inward until you can no longer breathe in. Exhale slowly and steadily so that all of the air escapes your lungs. Repeat these two more times.

Focus your attention on your body and your weight now. Visualize in your mind what you look like and try not to judge yourself too harshly. You are who you are, no matter what you look like or how you feel about that. Erase the tension and negativity from your mind; just be present with yourself right now.

Say to yourself,

"I am beautiful. I am strong. I can do this. I will lose weight, and I will not let anyone or anything stand in my way. The only opinion I will accept is what I think and feel about myself. At this moment and in my future moments, I believe that I am beautiful just the way that I am."

Let your breath suck in all these thoughts and have your mind believe everything you tell yourself as if it was your last wish on Earth.

Say to yourself

"I got this. I will not give up. I will achieve this, and I will make it to the finish line. I will conquer my fears and overcome every obstacle that stands in my way."

In the background, you hear a coach shout, "Ready, get set..." Bring your awareness to your breath again. Inhale deeply and as you breathe in, get yourself fully committed and ready to take your first step toward losing weight. "Go!" Breathe out and visualize your feet, taking that first, second, and third step forward. Feel the pressure of your body press down on your legs and carry you forward. You realize this is hard, but you don't give up. You continue to jog ahead. Repeat this – "I know I can, I know I can, I know I can. I won't give up; I can do this."

You are now coming up to a bicycle, and as you get on it, you feel the bike hold your weight. You will not fall. Put your feet on the pedals and start cycling.

Bring your attention now to your breath. You are breathing heavily, your heart is racing, your chest hurts, but it's a euphoric feeling. You feel free; you broke out of the cycle and crossed the finish line. As you take a look down your body, you notice your body has become thinner. There is a scale in front of you on the sidelines; you've lost ten pounds. The feeling you are experiencing at this very moment is breathtaking, so you want to try it again. Trust that your body knows you and what to do. Trust in yourself that you will get through this.

Five, four, three, two, one, and go! Let out your breath and feel your legs carry your ten-pounds-lighter body. This time it's a little more comfortable than the first round. Your breath quickens, and your heart speeds up. You can do this.

Say to yourself,

"I will complete this course. I am strong enough to conquer any barrier that stands in my way. This is hard, but nothing easy is worth doing. I got this."

151

In front of you now is a blow-up house with a wide opening. You crawl through this opening and are covered by colorful plastic balls. They are flying at you from all angles, and it becomes hard to see. Soon, you are swimming through these balls moving forward. You push these balls aside, and as you look up, you see another opening. "I got this,"
You say to yourself.

"I will make it through, and nothing can stop me now." As you reach the opening, you crawl through and are entirely on your stomach. You are in a narrow hole that you must army-crawl through to reach the end. Take in a deep breath now. Nothing scares you. Nothing can get to you. Imagine this hole the way everyone else bullied you or picked on you. You might have felt small, or enclosed, singled out, or trapped.

You have complete control. You can do this. You are coming closer to the light at the end now. Nothing can stop you. As you reach the end of the tunnel, you jump out and start doing jumping jacks and yell to the universe, "I did it!" You beat your fears, and you conquered the darkness, but your journey isn't over yet. On the right side of you is freshwater on the table with a scale right next to it. You down the water and step on the scale. You notice your weight dropped another ten pounds. As the euphoric energy escapes you, you feel happy and delighted.

As you look ahead of you, you see one more course twenty feet away and the finish line at the end. Take a step forward now. Walk or jog at your own pace. You got this. You have faced more difficult challenges before, so you are going to get through this one. Twenty steps later and you reach a potato sack, and five tires on the ground laid out in a straight line. You jump into the potato sack, and while holding it up, you jump into the first tire hole. Take a deep breath in, and now the second tire hole. Breathe out, jump into the third tire, now the fourth, and take your time. Breathe in and jump into the final tire.

As you jump out to finish, exhale slowly. You can feel your heart aching from the exercise. Pat yourself on the back; you are almost finished. On the left side of the track, you notice weight balls that attach to your ankles and two five-pound dumbbells. You connect the ankle weights, pick up the dumbbells in each hand, and look forward. The finish line is ten steps away. Take a deep breath in. "I'm almost there, and I won't give up." Breathe out and take your first step. The weight around your ankles was the same amount of weight you carried at the beginning of the race. You notice how much of a difference this is and never want to feel like this again. Take another step forward and feel the sweat drip down the back of your neck. Feel the exhaustion.

Now visualize your ideal weight. Let that be your motivation to continue. With every step, you become more and more tired. Your body becomes more and more exhausted, but you don't give up, you keep moving forward; the finish line just steps away now. Take a deep breath in, and there is no way you are giving up now. You are so close to your ideal weight. You have almost accomplished your goal. You hear the people on either side of you cheer you on. Yes! You crossed the finish line and felt that it was all worth it as you step onto that scale beside you. And right before your very eyes are the numbers you have wanted to see for so long.

You did it! Congratulations! You are now at your ideal weight. Visualize what this looks like and take in the excitement. Visualize what feeling you would experience after completing your goal. Stay relaxed at this moment for as long as you would like.

When you are ready, come back to the present moment. Bring your awareness to your breath. Move each finger and wiggle your toes. Feel good as you remember your visualization. You completed your goal, and you didn't give up. That's what you will choose to do in your waking life every day. Everyone has obstacles, but you have the willpower and now the skills to beat everyone that gets in your way. You may open your eyes now.

Chapter 29. More Scripts for Guided Meditation/Self Hypnosis

Natural weight loss meditation #1

Sit back, relax and close your eyes

Feel the tension on your forehead

Feel all the tension go away.

Feel this relaxation on your forehead

And in your eyes

And now your eyelids are getting heavy

So heavy that they don't even want to open, they are so relaxed

They might flutter a little.

But it's okay...

Feel how heavy they are.

Your mouth may even open a little

It's normal...

Relax with every breath you take,

You're so relaxed now

Having more relaxation with each deep breath, you are inhaling

Go into deep now and, breathe heavier as you go deeper

Now imagine this...

Imagine being in this wonderful and charming field

At the soles of your feet, there are a beautiful walkway and brick stairs

This leads to a very relaxing forest and danger -free forest

These steps will take you to a very deep state of deep hypnosis.

Get these steps together now.

While counting down from ten going to zero

Each problem will take you deep into where you are supposed to go

That's right, very good; it's going very well now.

10: step down

9: getting deeper

8: now down

7: even deeper

6: feeling very relaxed

5: Going deeper

4: you are now going into a state of deep and deep hypnosis

3: deepen

2: you are very relaxed that you can even move around, having that feeling of comfort. Very comfortable than ever, never felt before

1: you will now go to this wonderful place of tranquility and peace called deep and deep hypnosis.

0: continues to go very deep so relaxed and calm; go on and relax now, breathe with ease, and listening to light music as you enter the further.

Visualize a door

in front of you

It has a positive sign on it

the positive sign points out that you enter;

When you open the door, you look at the four steps

Descending to a room full of meters and dials on all the walls.

Go and step on those blocks, going down

Please note that all counters and dials look to continue indefinitely.

There are a lot of dials and meters

But when you take a glance, you see that each one is individually labeled.

A meter is labeled "metabolism."

One is labeled "cholesterol."

Another is labeled "blood pressure."

And another labeled " weight and body fat."

And while you look at billions and billions of quadrants and meters

You will understand that you are now in your mind's control room

You sit in the center of this control room, and there is a notebook called "perfect health."

In that notebook is your name

Go to that notebook

Take a look inside

Browse through words indicated there

Start to look that pages of this notebook have an image of each quadrant and a configuration in the quadrant;

It is representing good health for you.

Start scrolling through the pages

As you browse the notebook, you look at the mirror located at the corner of the place.

You approach the mirror

While you look at yourself in this mirror

Visualize the mirror manifesting all the variety of angles

In this very mirror, you will visualize a perfect reflection of you with the ideal size and weight you want to achieve.

Look at you from all angles

All seems at their proper place, those curves
Your clothes adapt perfectly to your body.

As you look at the mirror's reflecting the perfect beauty you possess,
Listen to your reflection by giving them these suggestions:
Starting today, I will chew my food slower and longer
Starting today, when I am sitting down to eat;
I will measure my hunger level on a scale of one to five
Zero is starving, and five are so full that I can't eat another bite.
Starting today, I will stop eating at 6 or 7.
Now I want to eat a healthy and fresh source of vegetables.
Keep in mind that your reflection reaches out to hold yours
When his hands come in contact, you are feeling an unconditional type
of love from you're the reflected version of you
Feel the deep love poured to your heart
And then look at the reflection reaching out your hand
When you go on and reaching your reflection;
Step forward in the reflection in the mirror become you
Indulge in how nice it is to become that reflection
Take yourself out of that mirror into a new life of vitality and health.
Go back to your perfect health control room
Start allowing yourself to make safe and moderate adjustments.
Start drawing your awareness to the inside your body and its sensation
As you feel, you begin to correct.
That's right...
Start feeling the sensations

Feel the ideal weight you want

Now your body is beginning to become the perfect size

Reaching the weight you want

I will count from one to five, and by doing so, you will wake up.

With every count, you'll make sure these suggestions are deep in your unconscious mind:

1: see the shape and size you want to be, which you are deserving of

2: feel great now that you know you have the control

3: you want healthy foods to help you weigh your ideal weight

4: you are no prepared to do whatever it takes to accomplish this and

5: open your eyes, fully awake, alert and bright, now fully awake.

That's right...

Fast weight loss meditation #2

Start by making yourself comfortable

Start settling in.

Stop worrying about how deeply you are relaxing and going into a trance

You don't even need to try.

Just listen...

Now, breathe deeply.

and other

Keep noticing your slow, steady breathing

Be aware of the feeling that the chest rises and falls

Now start feeling positive air pressure

With the breath coming

As you let the air out

You can also visualize that the air is safe,

Healing color when it goes inside your body and as it leaves.

It also guides you to a deeply relaxed state

Now you are relaxed...

Time to treat the part of yourself not wanting to lose weight.

Part of you can rebel against your target

That's it...

Yes, the one part of yourself not wanting to lose weight

Now you can confront that piece of you

Not as a rival or a victim.

But as a friend, you long to meet

This piece of you is hurting

Dismissed by others

Dismissed by you

And this is the moment of healing

Now is the time to have peace inside of you

Now you have the opportunity to reconcile

Slowly, consistently, and successfully reach your ideal weight

Let this happen...

Let these words go deep as you say you hear them

I'm sorry you're hurt.

You have been suffering hurt inflicted by other people

I have disregarded you

It's time for healing to take place

I would like you to have felt being adored and loved

Let's work together

Let's end this war

We can make peace. It depends on us.

Imagine making peace with yourself now.

And feel the healing energy going through your body.

By pooling their strengths and resources,

Heal your weaknesses and close the gap that has been in your soul,

It prevents you from fully embracing your healthiest sense of self.

You

are a genuine person

With all your talents and strength available to pieces of yourself.

Be confident of yourself

Show yourself in your feeling and thoughts

You'll soon know all the parts of yourself that align with the healthiest

version of you

mentally, Physically spiritually and emotionally

Nourishing food will have great taste

Food that is bad for you will taste, empty, fake, and lifeless.

You will have the motivation to move your body.

Invites a feeling of being vibrant of fitness and general well-being

Go ahead and have that peace you need internally

Show strength outwardly.

Begin to see weight loss come naturally.

Allow what you gained at this moment to be integrated into your whole being

And at the moment you select to imagine yourself in front of a mirror.

Imagine that you are in your favorite outfit.

With the exact weight you want

Feel awake relaxed and hopeful.

Imagine that your body weight begins to move towards the desired weight.

Now take your time...

With every count, you'll make sure these suggestions sink deep in your unconscious mind:

1: see yourself the size and shape you want to be, you deserve to be.

2: feel wonderful about yourself, finally knowing that you are in control

3: you want healthy foods to help you weigh your ideal weight

4: ready now to do whatever it takes to accomplish this

5: eyes open, fully awake, bright and alert, now fully awake.

That's right...

Guided Meditation for Self-Hypnosis #3

Please make yourself comfortable

Take a deep breath

Relaxing with every breath

You have a great feeling of relaxation now

Keep noticing your slow, steady breathing...

Pay close attention to the feeling that the chest rises and falls

With the breath coming

Feel that positive air pressure

Just relax...

Feel that your eyelids are becoming heavy

So heavy that they don't even want to open

But it's okay...

Now to decide the time to lose weight

Create an image in the mind of yourself in the future with your goal weight on that date.

I want you to see exactly how you will look.

See how happy you will be.

And imagine how happy you will feel.

Make the image big and bright.

You can feel that smile grow as you easily imagine

Easily reach your goal

See how compelling that image is to yourself.

It's time to visualize a picture that you are halfway to your dream

Visualize how great you are feeling, knowing that you are halfway to your goal.

Look how good you are.

See how much has improved since today.

I need you to visualize waking up tomorrow morning

Having an enormous amount of energy, realizing you are on your way to achieving your goal,

Knowing that the more you see your end goal, the easier it will be

Go effortlessly and get exactly what you want.

Now it's time for your unconscious part of beginning making changes

Imagine your goal and motivate yourself even more

Understand what it means to you now. Learn to enjoy exercise.

Look forward to getting around every day!

Eliminate you're eating compulsions

Eat healthily

Change your daily eating habits

Feel the sensations

Feel the perfect weight you want

Feel your body weight begin to move towards perfect size

Achieve the desired weight

I will count from numbers one to five, and by doing so, you will wake up.

With every count, you'll make sure these suggestions are deep in your unconscious mind:

1: see yourself the size and shape you want to be, you deserve to be.

2: feel wonderful about yourself, finally knowing that you are in control

3: you want healthy foods to help you weigh your ideal weight

4: ready now to do whatever it takes to accomplish this and

5: eyes open, fully awake, bright and alert, now fully awake. Straight.

Chapter 30. Daily routine

For your quick workout routine, walk up through the stairs at your workplace. Park your car at the farthest spot and trek all the way distance. Take your dog on a long walk. Participate in every way you can. That is the primary purpose of exercising. If you haven't done any workout or you couldn't get going in one moment, don't just hang up on it, just get back on schedule the following day.

Set a routine for everyday hypnosis meditation and affirmation for weight loss

If you're still doing some old-style aerobics' classes, then you could mix things up and try to take the latest gym class available. A number of the most preferred gym classes that you could take include indoor cycling, boxing-based programs, yoga classes acrobatics, and martial art. This will help you to be able to combat being bored, which is the main reason why you participate in emotional eating and quit exercising. Try always to drink a lot of water while exercising. Warm-up before exercising. If you haven't warmed up, then you have to get into the warming up routine before every exercise. Habitually do it to warm up. It isn't needed to do some warming up before any tough exercise, but by doing so, you'll be able to get your blood flowing, and you be are enabled in preparing yourself for any activity you will be doing

Standing Reach Stretch

One of the stretching exercises that you can do is the standing reach stretch. This stretch involves the upper body's movement. So start with your arms, keep your arms straight down, besides your bodies with your palms facing backward. Use one arm, raise it forward, and raise it up as

165

high as possible. Now tighten your abs and use the opposite arm to touch your shoulders and stretch across your chest slightly. Now maintain this stretch 10 to 30 seconds.

Repeat the same stretch with your arms reaching in the opposite direction. The neck stretches the chest and backstretch. Use your hands to grab the ends of a small towel in both hands. Now bring your arms to the chest level and slightly tuck on the ends of the towel and hold it for about 10 to 30 seconds.

Neck Stretch

Neck stretch is the upper-body stretch. This stretch is very good for golfers. Grab the end of a small towel with your end and slightly tuck them to the end of the wall.

The chest and Shoulders stretch

Now the next stretch is the chest and shoulder stretch. This stretch is great after swimming. So take your hands behind you, and hold the end of a towel at your hip. Now raise your chest high and raise your arms forward now hold the stretch for about 30 seconds.

Quadriceps Stretch

The next stretch is the quadriceps stretch. This stretch is good for runners, high-cut cyclists, and walkers. Sit behind the seat and grasp onto the chair for balance and support. Now take one hand and grab your other ankle. Gently push your foot forward towards your gluts. Do not tuck or slant forward but maintain your chest high-lifted. Now do this stretch for about 10 to 30 seconds. Now repeat the same thing on your other leg.

166

Standing Stretch for outer thigh

Go behind the seat and grasp the back of the chair for balance. Place one of your feet behind the chair and diagonally press your heels to the floor. Hold the stretch for about 30 seconds and put it doing using your other leg.

Tendon Stretch Arm's Length

The next stretch is the tendon stretch stand. Keep your length, about one meter behind the seat, and grasp onto the back of the chair supporting and balancing yourself. Now maintain your feet a few centimeters apart from your toes why you point your heels to the ground. Push your pelvis with care while bending the elbows, leaning forward. Now. Supporting yourself using your hands to the back of the seat. Now do this for about 30 seconds.

Standing stretch for shins

The next stretch the standing shin stretch. Stand at the back of a seat and grasp the back of the seat for balance and support. Bend your nails slightly and lift the toes of your feet off the ground while relaxing on the heels. Do this stretch for about 30 seconds.

The Hip Stretch

The next one is the hip stretch. Go behind the seat and grasp the back of the chair for balance and support while bending your nails across and intersect one of your ankles the opposite leg. Now sit back watch and hold it straight for about 30 seconds. Repeat this stretch, cross it to the other ankle over to the opposing knee.

Upper back Stretch and shoulder stretch

The next one is upper backstretch and shoulder stretch. This stretch is perfect for movements that need the upper body and bending movements. So to begin the stretch, stand behind the seat and grasp onto the back of the chair for support. Then take a step off from the seat until the arms are fully stretched. Now move and lean forward from your waist and stretch your shoulders forward, then hold onto the knee for about 30 seconds.

Try to stretch as many ways as you can; the more stretches that you do, the more likely, you will be to avoid tight muscles, prevent injuries, and feel better if your muscles are tight, patient with it. It will take some time for your muscles to go back to their normal length. Stretching throughout your life will help to reduce the effect of aging and will help me to lose weight and reduce the wear and tear of your joints and tissue. Studies have shown that it is possible to maintain your flexibility through a wide-stretching program that you can follow. You should remember that stretching is not a contest, you shouldn't compare yourself with other people because everybody is different. Some days you might be feeling bar where are some days you might feel tighter. Stay comfortably within your limits and allow the flow of your energy to come through you.

Abs

The first one is the abs. So grab a bubble chair or a dumbbell and then lie down on the back, while pointing your feet upright. Get the weight and stretch out your arms over it, and then contract your abdominal muscles while lifting the weight up facing the ceiling. Breathe out while moving up and breathe in a while, moving downward. Now you should remember not to do some bouncing on the ball. Moves slowly so that your muscles will be tightening enough as you do the whole rep, also try to bring your weight at an angle and strive to push the weight straight all perfectly vertical. Now the equipment that you need for this exercise are dumbbells and exercise balls, whereas the muscles that you are working out are the upper abdominal and the core muscles.

Chapter 31. Daily Weight Loss Script

This meditation is going to be focused on losing weight naturally. Listen to this directly or repeat the script in your own voice and use that to help guide you through the meditation. Find a comfortable position and begin when you are ready. Let these thoughts flow through your mind naturally, as if you were saying them.

I can feel each breath that enters and exits my body. It is so natural to feel myself breathing. I can feel my lungs expand, and my chest straighten as I am sitting comfortably, my shoulders relaxed. As the air gives me life, I feel connected to the earth. All that is living needs oxygen. Even fire needs oxygen.

I can see from the things that surround me that air is good. The air is healthy. The things that are naturally present and existing in my world are healthy. I am supposed to do what comes naturally.

The things that feel right are the ones that are the easiest. Getting healthier than how I now feel natural. It is what is easiest for me. When I feel the water, I feel natural. Drinking water, filling my body with what is natural, this all makes me feel healthy. When I am healthy, I am losing weight. My body is adjusting itself to its natural state, where it is supposed to be when I eat foods from the earth and exercise the way that I should.

There have been unhealthy measures I've considered, and maybe even taken, in the past. Some companies have convinced me to take drastic measures, through supplements and crash diets.

None of these measures worked for me. This is because of what I know now; the only way to lose weight is to do so naturally. When I have the ability to do this, I can do anything. Losing weight naturally is the only way to find success. All of the other methods haven't worked out for me because they weren't supposed to.

What I am supposed to do now is to lose weight healthily. I am going to make sure that I am eating the right foods and doing things that my body is supposed to do.

I forgive myself for hurting my body. I need to lose weight naturally because I don't want to suffer from any more pain. Any crash dieting only hurts other parts of my body. I need to take care of the skin I am in because it is the only one I will ever have. I deserve to treat my body right because I don't have any other options. This is going to be the method that helps me achieve my goals and takes me to a place that I have only fantasized about in the past.

I know now that I need to be healthy in order to live a long and happy life. Any shortcuts I take will only do just that – make things short. I do not want to live a short life. I want to live one that is long and happy. When I take care of my body, this is possible. I can live a free life where I don't worry about my health as much as I do now.

I deserve to eat healthy foods that make my body feel good. Going forward, everything good that happens to me is something that I deserve. I no longer want to punish myself for doing things that are natural.

I choose to eat healthily because it is what is going to make me feel good overall. I can allow myself to eat junk food occasionally, but I understand that eating healthy is the only long-term option that I have.

Exercising is good for my body because it helps it to become stronger. When I can get on the treadmill or workout, that is when I feel the most powerful. When I am aware of all the muscles in my body working together to take me to amazing places, I feel like I am in control of my life.

Being physically fit makes me feel strong physically, but especially mentally. I have confidence in my body. I hold myself right and with confidence. My posture shows that I love myself and that my body is healthy. I sit up straight and keep my legs stretched so that I am not forcing myself to have bad posture.

I want to be strong and healthy, so that it is easy to move around. I enjoy feeling physically fit so I can climb stairs and go for walks. When I am with other people, it is easier to be physically fit so we can do exercises together without me worrying about how I look or feel.

I can be more active with my friends and family when I am losing weight naturally. I broaden my options for activities when I am naturally losing weight because I know that I can do anything. I don't fear what might lie ahead.

Eating a natural diet will give me other health benefits besides just losing weight. I can reduce my risk of getting certain diseases and cancers when I make healthy choices. I accept that age will make it harder to maintain certain weights, but I will always practice healthy, natural habits because that is what matters the most.

If I am taking supplements, that will not help me for a long period of time. By losing weight naturally, I am able to show my body how much I love it. I am adjusting myself for the upcoming years so that I will have less to worry about.

It is peaceful knowing that I am going to lose weight naturally, in a way that won't hurt my body. I won't have to worry about having any other health concerns with my body when I know that I can lose weight naturally.

I can feel my breathing in a rhythmic pattern that helps to relax my mind, body, and soul. It feels so good, so natural to let the air travel in and out of my body. This breathing is going to help me in the future when it is time to exercise. I feel the air come into my body, and slowly leave. Each breath that I take reminds me that I am alive and that I deserve to live the best life possible.

It is time to become either focused or drift asleep now. As I count down from ten again, I will be out of this meditative state and back into the world that will help me to lose weight successfully. Ten, nine, eight, seven, six, five, four, three, two, one.

Chapter 32. Hypnotic Gastric Band

The Hypnotic Gastric Band is used in many national publications to help people lose weight. Many people find it. While we had always been a great success with my conventional hypnosis and coaching when people began to talk about hypnotic gastric bands, we were not sure about what to do.

What's the trick, then?

We all have strong belief systems, and we must brush our teeth every day, we must remember to buy the birthday cart our loved ones, we must go to bed before a certain amount of time so that on the next day we do not feel so tired.

If we think we have a smaller stomach that doesn't have enough calories to internalize it into our brains. What is hypnosis doing? We might talk Freudian and start with we'd, the ego and the superego, but for another time, we'll save that.

We are very open to suggestions, to new beliefs, when we have our eyes closed and comfortable, and we are in a place where we are not afraid to be honest (the therapist's office). We use our conscious minds when we are alive, to combat such things as a desire to avoid consuming the cream cake. Still, when we see that cake, the selfish part (say, we d) begins to excuse us, life "Go one treat, you deserve it," and thus our conscious "will power fails a little as though it is not fused when it is too much electrical power. Through calming the mind, we can reach the core belief structures that have established our values and beliefs over the years.

You will reinforce your confidence under hypnosis over and over until you have a strong belief that we should brush our teeth daily. Return to the gastric ribbon. With the Hypnotic Gastric Band, you reassure the consumer that his belly is low and that he cannot have enough food, but that will never be enough, in my opinion. You see that my technique is much more comprehensive than just making people think that they have tiny stomachs and that works.

Step 1— Knowing the person, their diet, their self-esteem, their training schemes, what motivates them, etc.

Step 2 — Make a connection and trust by a detailed discussion of issues in step 1.

Step 3-Coaching and CBT strategies to develop a plan that blends balanced food and exercise with a healthy social life.

Step 4— improve it by hypnosis

Step 5 — add gastric band by hypnosis.

Step 6-Feel good inside when the card tells how you changed somebody's life for the better. Beauty works, so if you're a therapist who wants to help others, my way of doing it is tried and checked.

If you're a person who has a great desire to lose weight, you have to try it out.

Hypnotherapy Gastric Band Hypnosis

If you are clinically obese-the BMI over 30-it is extremely optimistic about having a virtual gastric band that is fitted with the hypnoses-yes, hypnotherapy is the strongest all-round choice for weight loss.

I have run two successful weight loss programs together, and so many people with their weight problems have great experience-both have the same philosophies. Many people on their diet want the items they should not consume, or they return to their old ways after dieting and losing weight. Some of their diets may exclude many foods-leaving an unbalanced diet that stresses their liver and kidneys-which may be very harmful.

I think it is essential to make people have an awareness of how much to eat healthy foods and persuade them that it is less cost-effective to eat high-quality products than cheaper fatty sugar and salt-saturated ones–good food really does offer a better price for the buck. Won't you put paraffin into your petrol tank? To go further in this example for comfort eaters, would you not put fuel in the car if the oil light comes on? Yet the oil light is a sign that something is wrong, and the issue is not solved to put chocolate in your mouth. Comfort food addresses nothing but obesity.

Many of these issues are associated with psychological tension, lack of self-confidence, or childhood behaviors that are developed into poor eating patterns as they grow up. I say better waste bin pounds than waist pounds!

Hypnotherapy may address these problems–it offers methods for addressing anxiety and stress and a lack of trust, and it uses approaches such as regression to resolve psychological problems, which could result in an abusive food relationship. Another lady with 21 stones came, and when we dealt with her bullying problems, she started to lose weight quickly-something she had never been able to do! It was a dietary suggestion!

Furthermore, today, the U.S. Health Authority has added fat sugar and salt to junk food, which you can call "junkie" food, and the taste buds are addicted to this matter. If you've ever watched "supersize me," you know how dangerous it may be, especially when the quality of food is skewed towards junk food.

The food diary is another important weapon, recording what you consume, but also when and why you eat certain foods?

When obesity hits a BMI level of over 30, then some people have a very bad choice: they will have terrible health issues if they do not lose weight–they will have all the diets and drugs checked and failed, as all the underlying problems for overeating have not been dealt with. Sometimes they have the only choice of a gastric tape — the procedure can cost from £ 3,000 to £ 7,000 — in some situations, it can be risky — I have just had a client that has had multiple strokes, and two of them serious— complications for them are too big.

The combination of good nutritional advice and learning to eat properly and to cope with psychological problems will lead to a permanent loss of weight. Therefore, weight loss is much more likely when the virtual gastric band is placed under hypnosis using something like the HypnoGastricBand system. The system works for most people, and consumers have stated that they can not only see and observe the process painlessly but also sense it when it's activated. The discomfort passes quickly, people start to eat smaller portions, and like my other weight loss clients, they eat less, exercise more, and start to have food again.

The procedure of the stomach band is spoken of under hypnosis. As keyhole surgery, it is relatively simple-bind a band around the upper part of your stomach–the band can be tightened or loosened, and the golf ball made up part of the stomach means the hypothalamus, the appetites operator, informs you that you are complete-the food passes normally. The hypnotic gastric ribbon placed under hypnosis is the same as a real gastric ribbon. There are also weight loss programs with a BMI under 30, which do the same but do not suit the gastric band.

Chapter 33. Specific weight loss tips for women

Eat Healthy

Would it be advisable for you to start a better eating routine or create smart dieting propensities to get in shape? For some individuals, the main thing they consider with regards to weight reduction is that they ought to start eating better. In all actuality for long haul benefits, the propensity for eating nutritiously is a vastly improved alternative for a few reasons.

The very notice of "starting a better eating routine" infers that you will later fall off of that diet. That in that spot reveals to you that eating fewer carbs is a momentary way to deal with a way of life issue. Sure, craze diets may work for the time being, yet over the long haul, they, for the most part, don't give any genuine advantage. Individuals need to shed pounds and keep it off. By learning the best possible strategies for weight control and keeping up smart dieting propensities, you are substantially more liable to reach and remain at your ideal weight. Giving exceptionally nutritious foods in the best possible sums is the ideal approach to fuel your body and control your weight.

Many "prevailing fashion eats less" increase momentary fame for the straightforward explanation that they give present moment, quick weight reduction, these eating regimens are frequently founded on taking out some nutritious foods and supplanting them with shakes, caffeinated drinks or other enchantment elixirs, diet pills, high fiber blends or costly prepared dinners. Some of the time, definitely diminishing your calories is a piece of these weight control plans. It is imperative to recollect that your body is powered by the nourishment you eat. To work at an elevated level, be solid and enthusiastic, it is indispensable to supply your body with exceptionally nutritious foods. Expelling nutritious foods from your eating regimen in a hurry to get more fit can't insightful choice. At times quick weight reduction can accomplish more mischief than anything.

A great many people comprehend that your body's digestion is imperative to weight control. Think about your digestion as your degree of vitality use. Utilizing less energy can prompt weight gain since muscle to fat ratio is an abundance vitality that gets put away in fat cells. By diminishing weight too quickly it can really make your body hinder your digestion. This, thus, can make you sleeper weight after the underlying quick weight reduction of an eating routine. Known as the yo-yo impact, this is a main source of disappointment for people hoping to get thinner and keep it off. By joining appropriate dietary patterns and reasonable exercise, you can successfully keep up your digestion working at its legitimate level, which will help with controlling your weight. Muscle-fortifying activity, which straightforwardly expands your digestion, is significant, as is normal cardio aerobic exercise.

A couple of key focuses on appropriate eating ought to be remembered. Eating a few generally little estimated dinners and snacks for the duration of the day is a superior methodology than bigger, less continuous suppers. Try not to skip breakfast - it truly is the most significant dinner of the day. Eating normally keeps up your digestion. Select crisp foods and genuine items, including natural food sources, are vastly improved nourishment decisions than exceptionally handled, substance, and sodium-filled foods.

Numerous individuals believe that eating nutritiously is hard to achieve. The methodology one should take is to create good dieting propensities to get in shape, keep up legitimate weight, and augment your wellbeing. Propensities, both great and awful, are difficult to break. When you set up great dietary patterns, those propensities will be generally simple to keep up for the basic season; your eating techniques are only that - a propensity. Some portion of building up a decent nourishing project is figuring out how to basic food items look for good nourishment decisions. Most visits to the market lead you to similar paths and choosing similar nourishment things. By becoming accustomed to continually purchasing a choice of sound, nutritious foods, it will guarantee that you have these things in your home.

Another misinterpretation about appropriate eating is that nutritious foods are exhausting, tasteless, and not delicious. Nothing can be further from reality. Legitimate nourishment arrangement, cooking techniques, nutritious plans, and sound nourishment substitution can prompt some amazingly solid and delectable dishes.

With the best possible disposition towards your wholesome propensities, it very well may be enjoyment, sound, and delicious approach to legitimate weight control. The feared "starting a better eating routine" approach can stay away from as you create smart dieting designs on your approach to great wellbeing and legitimate weight reduction.

In the event that you really record what you are regularly eating, you presumably will drop your jaw with sickening apprehension. We never think to include the little tad portion size piece of candy here and the two treats to really observe the significant effect it is having on our weight control plans. The ideal approach to accomplish a solid way of life, to the extent our weight control plans go, is eating more products of the soil. We as a whole know it, so for what reason do we head for the potato chips aisle in the supermarket rather than the produce segment?

Essentially it comes down to this. Low-quality foods trigger our craving and leave us aching for additional. Ever wonder why eating one minimal honest Cheez-it prompts eating a large portion of a case? One taste triggers your body to need to continue eating. Presently in the event that you could condition yourself to do that with red grapes, we could accomplish that solid way of life. It might be hard to do, however, not feasible. Here are five different ways to condition yourself to settle on more beneficial nibble decisions.

Out Of Sight, Out Of Mind

If you don't have good nourishment in your kitchen, you won't eat it. It truly is that straightforward. I am the sort of individual who needs something to eat while I watch my daily film, and I will, in general, get the terrible stuff. The main occasions I don't is the point at which I cannot. Do your shopping for food directly after you have eaten an enormous supper so you won't be eager for awful foods, yet rather great food sources. Leave the store with no low-quality nourishment yet with plenty of products fresh. Your handbag and your tummy will thank you over the long haul.

Add Fruits And Vegetables To Your Dishes

Some of the time, it is difficult to plunk down with a couple of strawberries without the chocolate plunge; you desire something terrible. That is the trigger nourishment shouting to you; however, you need not answer. Cut the strawberries up and add them to a bowl of oat. Toss in a couple of blueberries and raisins. Simply make sure to utilize skim milk and keep the sugar in the cabinet. Organic product has enough normal sweetness without anyone else. Consider it characteristic treats.

When was the last time you are excited to eat carrot and celery sticks without plunging sauce? Likely never, yet that doesn't mean you never will. Add them to a little serving of mixed greens when you need a tad portion. No, you cannot suffocate it all in greasy blue cheddar dressing. That is a similar thing as plunge, is it not? A tad of vinaigrette dressing is the thing that your psyche ought to consider.

Make a Compromise

In the event that you are following the American Diet, your palette presently pines for high salt and high sugar foods. Stopping is never fruitful when it is done immediately. Individuals think they have to stop all the awful stuff at the same time and afterward three days after the fact they wear out and return to negative behavior patterns. Being sound can't pass up the foods you love.

On the off chance that you need pizza, eat a cat with a bowl of natural product serving of mixed greens rather than French fries. In the event that you need Cheeze-Its, eat a bunch with a bunch of grapes rather than

183

a large portion of the cheez-It box. Straightforwardness into it and gradually improve your dietary patterns.

Load up on Liquids

Commonly we mistake strive after thirst. You think you are hungry until you drink a decent, reviving glass of water. At that point, your stomach feels somewhat fuller, and you have not included more calories to your midsection line. On the off chance that you make sure to drink fluids on a regular basis, you will likely get yourself not in any event, thinking you are eager any longer.

So in light of that, whenever you fear to request an excess of fettuccine Alfredo at your preferred Italian eatery, drink a tall glass of water before you request. You may want to pass that for a pleasant fresh plate of mixed greens with shrimp or chicken.

Take A Supplement

Once in a while, we get going in our lives and may have the best expectations to eat healthily; however, we cannot generally find solid foods to eat. Most candy machines don't offer carrot and celery sticks, shockingly. One route around this is to take a day by day supplement that gives all of you the sustenance you would get on the off chance that you ate heaps of products of the soil. This doesn't mean you should take them and keep eating giggles bars throughout the day, as you may have guessed. Garbage is still garbage.

Eating foods grown from the ground may not be something you are utilized to, however simply like whatever else, it takes some becoming accustomed to. Utilize the tips above to make progress simpler, yet don't take on a similar mindset as a con artist. Con artists never succeed, and in the event that it was simple, everybody would stroll around in very good shape. Carrying on with a sound way of life implies settling on solid decisions. The more you are able to do it, the more benefits you will be.

Chapter 34. All About Hunger

We will look at the different types of hunger and how you can tell them apart. This will help you to distinguish when you are hungry and when you may be turning to food to soothe your emotional state.

Real Hunger vs. Perceived Hunger

It can be difficult to tell sometimes when we are really hungry, and when we may be feeling as though food will make us feel better emotionally. Real hunger is when our body needs nutrients or energy and is letting us know that we should replenish our energy soon. This happens when it has been a few hours since our last meal when we wake up in the morning, or after a lot of strenuous activity like a long hike. Our body uses hunger to signal to us that it is in need of more energy and that if it doesn't get it soon, it will begin to use our stored energy as fuel. While there is nothing wrong with our body using its stored fuel, it can be used as a sign to us that we should eat shortly in order to replenish these stores.

Perceived hunger is when we think we are hungry, but our body doesn't actually require any more energy or for the stores to be replenished. This can be because our brain notices that it is the time of day when we would normally eat. Even if we have just eaten a short time before, when we are feeling stressed or anxious, and our body isn't sure how to soothe this, we think that food may help. When our emotional state makes us crave comfort and good feelings, we—our brains—know that we can get this from certain foods like sugary or fatty ones.

How to Tell the Difference Between Real Hunger and Perceived Hunger

When we feel hungry, there are several questions we can ask ourselves to determine whether we are hungry and in need of sustenance, or we are hungry because of an emotional need. Below, I have listed the questions to ask and what they can tell us about our hunger.

1. When did I last have a meal?

We want to ask ourselves this question because if we had a full meal less than two or three hours ago, it is likely that we are not experiencing actual hunger. The hunger is coming from something else like an emotional need or boredom.

2. How hungry am I?

Go within and ask yourself how hungry you are. While you don't want to wait until you are absolutely starving and light-headed to eat, you want to be hungry enough. If you are not quite at a level where you could eat a meal, you probably aren't hungry enough to eat just yet.

3. Am I still hungry now?

If you feel famished, drink water. Wait for 15 minutes and assess if you are still hungry afterward. If you are not, you could have just been hungry because of your emotional state.

4. Was there a change in my emotional state just previously?

Sometimes, we will feel the need or the compulsion to eat right after we get some bad news or have an upsetting thought or conversation. Ask yourself if you felt the feeling of hunger directly after one of these occurrences or something that you know to be a trigger for your emotional hunger. If something like this has just happened, you may not have connected them as being related. By taking a minute to recognize this, you can decide that you may not actually be hungry and address the emotional issue instead.

Emotional Hunger Isn't Satiated With Food

5. Do I feel hungry again right after eating?

If we begin to eat or have a snack when we feel emotional hunger, you may feel good right afterward, but shortly after, it will not be resolved. This is another way to find out whether you are actually hungry or not. If you do decide to eat something and shortly after you feel hungry again, you were likely not hungry for food but had an emotional need instead. Since this emotional need could not be resolved with food, you feel famished and crave that positive feeling you get right after eating once again a short time later.

6. Do I feel guilty about eating?

If we eat when we are hungry, and after we feel satisfied and ready to continue on with our day, we will not feel any sense of guilt or shame about it since we were fueling our bodies. However, if we ate when we had a craving, and we felt hunger, but it was an emotional need telling us we were hungry, we may feel guilty or ashamed afterward about having eaten. This feeling can indicate that we were not really hungry but that we were trying to fill a void that was not filled by eating food.

The reason that hunger doesn't become improved or disappear after eating is that the body craves food for that positive feeling when getting after we eat. Like we talked about at the initial part of this guide, eating certain foods or chemicals in food instead makes us feel rewarded and

188

happy temporarily because of the reaction in our brain that is similar to taking a drug. Our mind enjoys this feeling, and it helps to lift our mood or take our mind off of our emotional turmoil for the time being. The problem is that when these rewarding and positive feelings are gone because the chemicals have gone away, we return to feeling the way we did beforehand. The only way to truly resolve our emotions or feel better about something is to face them head-on. Trying to solve them by other means like eating or distracting ourselves will only work in the short term and will leave us feeling the exact same way after the distraction is gone.

How to Eat

We will now look at some methods to improve our eating habits in order to make them healthier for us. When you ask yourself all of the above questions, and you determine that you are in fact hungry, there are ways to eat to ensure that you are making the most of the time that you are eating, while also getting all of the nutrients that you need when you are eating. We will talk about something called mindful eating. Mindful eating is when you really get into the moment, instead of being distracted by everything that is going on in your mind. If you are feeling down emotionally when you do decide that it is time to eat, you may be focused on your emotional state and not really tasting or enjoying the food that you are eating. By practicing mindful eating, you will be present in your eating experience. When you go to eat, do so sitting down on a chair with your food on a table in front of you. This will help with digestion and help you to form a routine around eating. Being sure to eat mindfully and without distraction will help you to digest better as well, which will help you to get all the nutrients you need from your food. Before you take a bite of your food, notice the smells of the food you are about to eat. Notice how it looks- the colors and textures. As you put food in your mouth, feel the textures of the food on your tongue. Notice all of the flavors that you are tasting and the feeling that they bring to your mouth. Notice how it feels when you chew the food- how it feels on your teeth and your cheeks. Doing this with every bite will bring you into the moment and ensure that you are consciously eating every time that you eat. Consciously eating will make you more aware of everything that you put into your mouth, and focusing on the experience of eating can help you to have fewer cravings and less desire to eat in between meals. Try practicing this every time you eat.

When to Eat

we want to eat when we are hungry, but not when we are ravenous. If we are only mildly hungry, we can likely stand to wait for a little bite to eat. As a rule of thumb, when you start to become mildly hungry, begin to prepare your meal so that by the time you finish, you are the perfect level of hungry as you sit down to eat. If we do this in the future and not now, the way we eat can be absolutely ravenous, we will have let our blood sugar drop to quite a low level. We will likely have begun to get light-headed, irritable, and have some difficulty with decision making. If you feel like this when you are starting to eat, you will want to make a note to eat a bit earlier next time. The sweet spot is about a level 5 of hunger on a one to ten scale.

How Much To Eat

It can be hard to know how much to eat and when you have had enough without going to the point where you have eaten too much and feel completely full. This part includes some tips on how much to eat so that you can begin to tell how much is the right amount for you.

When we eat, it takes about twenty minutes for the hormone in our bodies that tells us that we are full to reach our brain. Our stomach is signaling our brain that we are hungry, and that signal takes about twenty minutes to reach the brain. Thus, we want to make sure that we eat slowly so that we can tell when we are full. If we eat very quickly, by the time we get the signal that we are full, we will have already eaten much more than we may have needed. Mindful eating will help you to eat slower than you normally might as you will be paying attention to each bite that you take. When you feel like you may be satiated, stop eating and wait for about twenty minutes. You will likely feel full then, but if not, you can always eat a bit more then.

Before you eat, drink a glass or so of water. This will help you to eat just the right amount and not too much, as this will help you to have something in your stomach already. This will also help with your digestion as the water will help everything to move smoothly along your digestive tract.

Chapter 35. Bonus Hypnosis: Maintaining Weight Loss

Hello, and welcome to your hypnosis weight loss session " Maintain weight loss and avoid yo-yo dieting with healthy eating habits" that will support your determination to lose weight and develop healthy eating habits, effortlessly, and as easily as possible. This session is hypnotic in nature, and it can easily put you in a state of relaxation and absorb your conscious attention inside. Please do not listen to this session while driving or operating any machinery or at any other time, which requires your full awaken attention.

I will guide you through this wonderfully relaxed experience and an amazing journey of discovering the inner strength and resources that will help you energize your inner will power so you can naturally start losing weight while enjoying the process of change.

This hypnosis session for weight loss is designed to introduce you to the Intermittent Fasting Strategy. We, as human beings, are not created to eat all the time. We need to burn that food by being active. Intermittent fasting is a great way to teach your body to burn food, rather than storing it. Intermittent fasting is also a great way to burn more fat when there is no food to burn. The effects of fasting only start to happen after 16 hours, and having in mind that we sleep for eight hours a day makes Intermittent fasting much easier to do because achieving a goal of eight hours of fasting is very easy. Everything else you must understand about this type of diet is that it is completely natural and completely free. All you have to do, in the beginning, is to choose which meal you are going to skip. Is it easier for you to skip breakfast, or is it easier for you to skip dinner? This strategy will help you always maintain your weight loss and develop healthy eating habits.

Let us start your weight loss hypnosis session and program your mind naturally develops healthy eating habits by implementing an intermittent fasting strategy...

Find a comfortable place to sit or lie down as you prepare yourself to go on a wonderful journey of increased relaxed awareness, tranquility, and peace. And the greatest thing about this journey is that you can do it anytime you want because you will remember how to go into relaxation... effortlessly... now… and every time you want to relax...

Your journey to develop a new and more supportive strategy for your weight loss begins by consciously choosing and instructing your body and mind to relax... by simply becoming aware of your breathing.

Notice the natural flow of your breath going in and out… there is no need to do anything… no need to change your breathing in any way, simply observe your body breathes.

Passively observe with your relaxed awareness your breath flowing gently in and out of your body… making you feel so relaxed deeper and deeper… with each breath you take…your breath takes you ...deeply... and calmly… into the most relaxing state of mind… each time you become aware of your breathing…

Feel the gentle rise and fall of your chest and abdomen… gently rising and falling with each relaxing breath in… and with each relaxing breath out… and as you feel this gentile rise and fall of your chest and abdomen... go even deeper into relaxation... that's right all the way down... completely relax and let go...

How is that relaxed awareness of your breathing affecting other parts of your body that are getting relaxed now... notice how much more you are getting relaxed right now when you become aware of your legs becoming relaxed... and even more relaxed when you pay attention to your toes... feet... calves... knees... thighs... all getting even more relaxed now...

And what about your fingers and palms... notice how much more you are getting relaxed as your awareness travels up from your fingertips and palms... to your forearms... arms and shoulders... your neck and back... all getting even more relaxed now...

All the muscles on your forehead.... all the tiny muscles around your eyes... and all the muscles around and inside your mouth including your tongue... all getting relaxed now...

Feel that pleasant tingling sensation of relaxation in every cell... making you even more relaxed... and because all your cells are connected... and can instantly share the same experience of comfort... and relaxation... that means... all other cells in your body can instantly relax in the same way right now... making your entire body completely relax right now...

That pleasant rhythm of tranquility and peace... inside your mind... is sending the signal to all the cells in your body... relax... connect with yourself... starting from your head and face... notice how this signal travels down your neck... filing every cell with relaxation... down your shoulders and arms... the pleasant tingling sensation of comfort... your chest... back... and stomach... know how to relax... just by listening to my voice... allowing the signal of relaxation to keep spreading down your

194

legs and feet and all the way back to your head... creating that continuous cycle of tranquility and peace inside your body right now... perfectly aligned with relaxing rhythm of your breathing.

In a moment, I am going to start counting down from ten to one. When you hear me utter "one," you will find yourself in a safe place, perhaps your favorite room, and you will be ready to install intermittent fasting strategy into your life... and always maintain your weight loss with healthy eating habits...

As you are now connected to your higher consciousness... use this moment to choose the option that is best for you... choose which meal you would feel happy to skip... is it breakfast or is it your dinner... choose the meal that allows you to have at least 14 hours between your last and initial meal...

Have you decided? Excellent, let us continue to deepen your relaxation Starting the countdown now... ten... nine... choosing one meal to skip every day... eight... seven... getting ready to install intermittent fasting strategy into your life... six… five… visualize your favorite save place... four... three... completely relaxed now... two... one... you are at your favorite safe place feeling safe and secure... free of all worries... ready to install intermittent fasting strategy and maintain your weight loss with healthy eating habits…

And as you do that and feel completely relaxed in your favorite safe place... I would like you to imagine a big screen in front of you... just like a movie theatre... and on that screen Imagine how would you look like in the future when you decide to do Intermittent Fasting strategy right now?... Think of all supportive actions that you need to take during everyday life for you to start naturally developing a healthy eating habit of intermittent fasting and maintain your ideal weight…

You already choose which meal you are going to skip every day as long as you are doing implementing intermittent fasting strategy... and that means you already choose two meals that are most important to you during the day...

Perhaps you would drink two or three extra glasses of water to hydrate yourself and compensate in the beginning until your body adjusts to this change... and perhaps you would allow yourself plenty of time to have a good night's rest when you go to sleep...

As you look at yourself on that screen imagine all the supportive actions you are taking to maintain your weight loss goals... imagine your stomach shrinking and having space only for two meals... and when you see yourself feeling lighter... being in control... and naturally developing healthier eating habit... imagine stepping into that screen so you can test and experience all these supporting actions and benefits of intermittent fasting...

Step into that screen... and experience how good you feel by limiting the amount of time each day that you allow yourself to eat... and notice how easier it is for you to maintain your ideal weight like this…

Become aware that a few extra glasses of water are giving you extra energy... and all of this combined together allows you to fall asleep more easily...

As you accept and take supportive actions for your weight loss plan... slowly step out of the screen... and come back to your favorite safe place... preserving all the learnings... and developing new and healthier behavior...

From now on, you are managing your daily food consumption and allowing your body to burn food and fat for your maximum benefit, health, and energy levels.

Do this now, preserve all the learnings and develop new and healthier behavior as I count down from ten to one. When you hear me utter" one," you will have everything that you need to make this work for you, so you can start maintaining your ideal weight naturally and easily...

Ten... nine... eight... preserving all the learnings... seven... six... five... accepting and taking new actions to maintain your ideal weight... four... three... your decision to live a healthier life is getting stronger and stronger... two... slowly starting to come back... one... allow your yourself to use Intermittent Fasting strategy naturally... and as soon as you are ready to open your eyes… become fully awake and alert in perfect health ready to implement your new behavior develop healthy eating habits.

Conclusion

Congratulations on getting to the end of the book. If you have been struggling to lose weight, you do not have to anymore. With the information you have gained from here, you can now embark on your weight loss journey with boldness because you know, this time, you will succeed. You can be sure that your efforts will not go in vain, far from it. This time you will achieve your goals and progressively become the person that you have always wanted to be.

Perhaps you have been yo-yo dieting, and every plan you engage in fails. By understanding the reasons, you overindulge is one of the best ways to begin this journey. Hypnotism is a great way to address any underlying issues that may be causing you to overeat and gain weight.

Hypnosis for weight loss is one of the best ways to lose weight. You will be able to get rid of it, and most importantly, you will gain the ability to control the way you eat. Keep in mind, this also can be helpful in reducing stress, and you can control the way you perceive things as well. It's a way to change the overall outlook of life, and it's also a great way to allow yourself the ability to achieve a good life that is full of happiness. You will be able to lose that unwanted weight, which begins with your capability in working your own hypnosis for losing weight

In this, you have also realized apart from going to see a professional hypnotist, and one can be able to self-hypnotize. You can do this to aid you in controlling the portions you eat.

At the end of it all, it is about eating consciously. Adapting mindful eating habits will help you maintain a healthy lifestyle even after reaching your goal weight. As you purpose to eat more attentively, be sure to engage a hypnotist that you can trust to take you through the journey. If you choose to self-hypnotize, you do not have to procrastinate anymore, download an app to help you and start your journey today.

Always remember calories and your consumption, as well as spending on them. Start physical exercises and control your portions to cut down on your calorie consumption. As such, this process does not have to be stressful. Far from it. It simply needs to be a routine that you can focus on so that it feels right for you.

Take every day of your days to celebrate your achievements because these achievements are what piles up to massive victory. Make a list of things you desire to change when you get healthy, and they may be small size-clothes, being able to accumulate enough energy, participating in your most loved sports you have been admiring for a more extended period, feeling self-assured. Make these tips your number one source of empowerment; you will end up completing your hypnosis sessions even without noticing. Do remember that your self-hypnosis plan should include suggestions that are more relevant to your relationship with food. This way, you could train your unconscious to slow down its automatic responses, while providing the unconscious with new and more useful ways to handle stress and emotions.

Once again, thank you for choosing this book. There are plenty of other options out there. By choosing this book, you have given us the motivation we need to continue doing our best to help others improve their lives and their wellbeing.

CPSIA information can be obtained
at www.ICGtesting.com
Printed in the USA
BVHW090849140621
609525BV00002B/128